MCQs in Applied Basic Sciences
For the Primary FRCS

K.M. Mokbel
Senior House Officer
Orthopaedic Surgery and Trauma
The General Infirmary
Leeds, UK

Presented as a service to medical education by

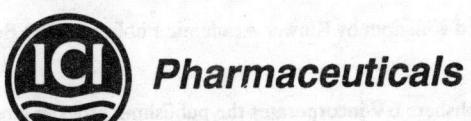

Pharmaceuticals

KLUWER ACADEMIC PUBLISHERS
DORDRECHT / BOSTON / LONDON

Distributors

for the United States and Canada: Kluwer Academic Publishers, PO Box 358, Accord Station, Hingham, MA 02018-0358, USA
for all other countries: Kluwer Academic Publishers Group, Distribution Center, PO Box 322, 3300 AH Dordrecht, The Netherlands

British Library Cataloguing in Publication Data

Mokbel, K. M. (Kefah M)
MCQs in applied basic sciences for the primary FRCS.
I. Title
616.0076

ISBN 0792389948

Copyright

© 1992 by Kluwer Academic Publishers

All rights reserved. No part of this publication may be reproduced, stored in a retrieval system, or transmitted in any form or by any means, electronic, mechanical, photocopying, recording or otherwise, without prior permission from the publishers, Kluwer Academic Publishers BV, PO Box 17, 3300 AA Dordrecht, The Netherlands.

Published in the United Kingdom by Kluwer Academic Publishers, PO Box 55, Lancaster, UK.

Kluwer Academic Publishers BV incorporates the publishing programmes of D. Reidel, Martinus Nijhoff, Dr W. Junk and MTP Press.

Printed and bound in Great Britain by Billings, Worcester.

Contents

Foreword	iv
Introduction	v
Acknowledgements	vi

Anatomy (including histology, embryology, and medical imaging)
    Questions   1
    Answers   24

Physiology and Biochemistry
    Questions   44
    Answers   61

Clinical Pharmacology
    Questions   73
    Answers   78

General and Systemic Pathology
    Questions   82
    Answers   91

Microbiology
    Questions   98
    Answers   103

Clinical Immunology
    Questions   108
    Answers   110

Haematology
    Questions   112
    Answers   114

Clinical Chemistry
    Questions   116
    Answers   119

Foreword

Multiple choice questions (MCQs) in medical and surgical examinations are now a new phenomenon. They have the advantage of testing knowledge rather than its presentation. However, although practice is the norm for essay questions and the viva-voce parts of examinations, it is equally crucial when dealing with MCQ papers where performance and examination outcome can be optimised.

As well as improving examination technique, practising MCQs also has the advantage of testing knowledge after a period of study, reinforcing knowledge gained as well as testing its acquisition, and, perhaps most importantly at what is to everyone a stressful time, providing reassurance that progress is being made.

This book provides a wealth of practice questions to serve these aims, although it should be remembered in using any such book that some questions will be more relevant than others to any examination and the First Part of the Fellowship is no exception to this principle.

Robert Ham
Consultant Vascular and General Surgeon
The Royal London Hospital
London E1

December 1991

Introduction

The MCQ format as part of examinations has come to stay. In an essay assessment, the examiner has to search the paragraphs for relevant facts and opinions and the examinee can take cover behind the smoke-screen of language. No such cover is provided by multiple choice questioning which not only allows electronic marking but also offers the candidate a fine stone to sharpen the knife of his knowledge.

The stimulus for writing this book came from the major changes in the FRCS examination which took place in England in September 1990. In the 'old' Primary FRCS examination many of the questions were not clinically relevant. Almost all the questions in the new Applied Basic Science part of the examination have a clinical bias. This new change has been reflected in this book in that almost all the questions have surgical relevance. Explanations to the answers have also been provided to make the MCQ exercise a more useful means of learning.

How to use the book

Each question has a main stem followed by five items, each of which must be identified as true (T) or false (F) or 'don't know'. In the exam a correct response gains one mark and an incorrect response is penalized by the deduction of one mark. The 'don't know' response gains nothing. The candidate is advised not to spend more than 2 minutes per question. A score of 50% is regarded as satisfactory.

MCQ terminology

'usually' = more than 50%
'rarely' = less than 5%
'never' = 0%   } these terms are not used
'always' = 100%   } in good MCQs
'characteristic' = refers to a feature which if absent would cause the diagnosis to be in doubt
'pathognomonic' = refers to a feature which is found in that disorder and no other
'associated' = more frequent than by chance
'the majority' = >60%

KM Mokbel
June 1991, London

Acknowledgements

Mr RJ Ham, Consultant in Vascular and General Surgery, The Royal London Hospital

Dr M Boyle, Senior Registrar in Morbid Anatomy, The Royal London Hospital

Dr BJ Houghton, Consultant in Clinical Chemistry, The Royal London Hospital

Dr E Shaw, Consultant and Lecturer in Microbiology, The Royal London Hospital

Professor D Vere, Professor in Clinical Pharmacology and Therapeutics, The University of London

Dr N Yeatman, Consultant and Lecturer in Clinical Immunology, The Royal London Hospital

The figures listed below have been redrawn from the following books, with the kind permission of the publishers:

Figure 4a: from Cuschieri A. Essential Surgical Practice. Bristol, John Wright [now Butterworth-Heinemann].

Figures 5, 6 and 7: from Snooks SJ, Wood RFM. Fundamental Anatomy for Operative General Surgery. Heidelberg, Springer-Verlag.

Figure 17a: from Blandy J. Lecture Notes in Urology. Oxford, Blackwell Scientific Publications

Anatomy (including histology, embryology, and medical imaging)

1. When performing an appendicectomy through the gridiron incision the surgeon will encounter

    A. the fibres of the external oblique muscle lying perpendicular to the line of incision
    B. the fibres of the internal oblique and transversus abdominis lying almost in a transverse direction
    C. Scarpa's fascia deep to the external oblique apeneurosis
    D. the trasversalis fascia fused to the peritoneum
    E. numerous communications between the appendicular artery and the ileal arteries

2. The great saphenous vein

    A. passes behind the medial malleolus
    B. joins the femoral vein about 3.5 cm below and lateral to the pubic tubercle
    C. usually lies behind the superficial external pudendal artery
    D. at the level of the saphenous opening, it receives fewer tributaries than the femoral vein
    E. has more deep perforators below the knee than in the thigh

3. The following statements refer to the postero-anterior plain radiograph of the skull

    A. the maxillary and ethmoidal air sinus produce a composite shadow
    B. the petrous parts of the temporal bones are superimposed on the lower halves of the orbits
    C. the film cassette is positioned behind the head when the X-ray is taken
    D. the coronoid and lambdoid sutures may be seen
    E. the atlanto-axial joint can be seen

4. When exposing the popliteal artery as part of an exploration of the popliteal fossa the surgeon will find the following relations

    A. the tibial nerve lies deep to the artery
    B. the popliteal vein lies between the popliteal artery and tibial nerve
    C. the artery lies on the popliteal ligament of the knee joint
    D. the tendon of semitendinosus lies lateral to the artery
    E. the peroneal nerve lies lateral to the artery

5. The left ureter

A. passes anterior to the fossa intersigmoidea
B. depends on its sympathetic innervation for its transport function of urine
C. receives its blood supply within the pelvis from the lateral side
D. crosses anterior to the left uterine artery about 2 cm lateral to the cervix
E. remains attached to the undersurface of the peritoneum when the latter is reflected at surgery

6. Regarding the anatomy of the pelvis

A. the middle rectal arteries run on the inferior surface of the levators ani muscles
B. the medial umbilical ligament represents the distal segment of the umbilical artery
C. most of the lymphatic drainage of the pelvic viscera reaches the inguinal lymph nodes
D. the nerves comprising the sacral plexus lie on the iliacus muscle
E. the obturator nerve gives off no branches to the pelvic viscera and muscles

7. The following refer to the femur

A. the neck normally makes an angle of 160° with the long axis of the shaft in a healthy middle-aged man
B. the intertrochanteric crest connects the two trochanters anteriorly
C. the shaft usually shows a forward convexity
D. the psoas muscle is attached to the greater trochanter
E. the two heads of the gastrocnemius muscle arise from the condyles of the femur

8. With respect to the blood supply to the femoral head

A. the obturator artery supplies the head via a branch which ascends through the femoral neck
B. the blood supply from the branch of the obturator artery is the most important item
C. the medial circumflex femoral artery supplies the head via branches that ascend along the neck deep to the synovial membrane
D. extracapsular fractures of the femoral neck severely damage the blood supply to the head
E. displaced subcapital fractures of the femoral head seriously damage the blood supply to the head

ANATOMY

9. A complete division of the femoral nerve results in

    A. foot drop
    B. paraesthesia of the lateral aspect of the foot
    C. failure of knee extension
    D. sensory loss over the medial part of the lower leg
    E. failure of adduction of the thigh at the hip joint

10. An injury to the ulnar nerve at the wrist results in

    A. wasting of the thenar eminence
    B. clawhand
    C. loss of the pincer-like action of the thumb and index finger
    D. sensory impairment over the palmar surface of the medial 1½ fingers
    E. wasting of the 2nd lumbrical muscle

11. With respect to surface anatomy

    A. the greater trochanter normally lies about 1 inch below a line joining the anterior superior iliac spine and the iliac tuberosity
    B. the lower orifice of the femoral canal lies below and lateral to the pubic tubercle
    C. the angle of Louis lies at the level of T2 vertebra
    D. the first rib lies deep to the clavicle and cannot be palpated
    E. the cricoid cartilage lies at the level of C6 vertebra

12. With respect to the knee joint

    A. the anterior half of the medial meniscus is relatively more mobile than the posterior half
    B. the medial meniscus is attached to the superficial fibres of the medial collateral ligament
    C. the suprapatellar bursa almost always communicates with the knee joint
    D. the tibia subluxates posteriorly when the posterior cruciate ligament is torn
    E. the central part of the meniscus is more vascular than its periphery

13. When performing a cholecystectomy the surgeon usually finds that

    A. the transverse colon lies anterior to the gallbladder
    B. the second part of the duodenum lies posterior to the gallbladder
    C. the cystic artery arises from the left hepatic artery
    D. the body of the gallbladder lies in direct contact with the visceral surface of the liver
    E. the right hepatic artery passes behind the common hepatic duct

14. With respect to inguinal hernias

A. the sac of a direct hernia bulges lateral to the inferior epigastric artery
B. the neck of an indirect hernia lies lateral to the inferior epigastric artery
C. direct hernias are commoner than indirect ones
D. the direct variety is commoner in older men
E. an indirect hernia is more likely to strangulate than a direct hernia

15. The structures of the spermatic cord include

A. the testicular artery
B. sympathetic fibres from the aortic sympathetic plexus
C. the cremasteric artery
D. the ilio-inguinal nerve
E. the testicular veins

16. The following statements refer to the inguinal canal

A. the posterior wall is formed by transversus abdominis
B. the canal allows the passage of the round ligament of the uterus to the labium majus
C. it transmits the ilio-hypogastric nerve
D. the superficial ring lies directly anterior to the deep ring in the newborn
E. on coughing, the canal becomes almost closed

17. The following refer to the inguinal canal

A. the medial part of the inferior wall is formed by the lacunar ligament
B. the superior wall is formed by the lowest fibres of external oblique
C. the posterior wall is re-inforced in its lateral third by the conjoint tendon
D. the anterior wall is re-inforced in its lateral third by the fibres of origin of internal oblique
E. the deep inguinal ring lies medial to the inferior epigastric vessels

18. With reference to the shoulder joint

A. the axillary nerve lies immediately below the humeral head
B. the rotator cuff passes between the coraco-acromial arch above and the humeral head below
C. posterior dislocation of the shoulder accounts for only about 3% of shoulder dislocations
D. internal rotation of the humerus increases the range of abduction at the gleno-humeral joint
E. an axillary approach is usually adopted to perform a shoulder arthroplasty

ANATOMY

19. The following structures lie within the parotid gland

　　A.　parotid lymph nodes
　　B.　the external carotid artery
　　C.　the external jugular vein
　　D.　the facial nerve
　　E.　the retromandibular vein

20. The thyrocervical trunk usually

　　A.　arises from the second part of the subclavian artery
　　B.　lies directly anterior to the stellate ganglion
　　C.　gives off the suprascapular artery
　　D.　gives off the deep cervical artery
　　E.　gives off the superior intercostal artery

21. When exploring the wrist the following structures are found to lie superficial to the flexor retinaculum

　　A.　the ulnar nerve
　　B.　the ulnar artery
　　C.　the median nerve
　　D.　the palmar cutaneous branch of the ulnar nerve
　　E.　flexor digitorum superficialis

22. The thyroid gland

　　A.　arises from the same branchial pouch as the upper parathyroid glands
　　B.　is separated from the strap muscles by the pretracheal fascia
　　C.　the middle thyroid vein courses laterally to drain into the internal jugular vein
　　D.　the upper parathyroid glands usually lie posterior to the gland and above the inferior thyroid artery
　　E.　in thyroidectomy, the recurrent laryngeal nerve is frequently damaged when ligating the superior thyroid artery

23. In radical neck dissection, the following structures are usually removed or sacrificed

　　A.　deep cervical lymph nodes
　　B.　spinal accessory nerve
　　C.　internal jugular vein
　　D.　mandibular branch of the facial nerve
　　E.　cervical sympathetic chain

24. With respect to the blood supply of the thyroid gland

A. the superior thyroid artery arises from the internal carotid
B. the superior thyroid artery descends to the upper pole of the thyroid lobe accompanied by the external laryngeal nerve
C. the thyroid ima, when present, may arise from the aortic arch
D. the inferior thyroid artery is closely related to the recurrent laryngeal nerve
E. the inferior thyroid veins drain into the left internal jugular vein

25. Damage to the sympathetic nerves from the thoracolumbar outflow (T11 to L2) will disturb the function of the

A. detrusor muscle
B. bladder neck
C. trigone
D. external sphincter
E. seminal vesicles

26. Branchial fistula

A. lies below the 3rd branchial arch
B. passes between the internal and external carotid arteries
C. shows a familial tendency
D. may have a muscular coat
E. is lined with squamous epithelium throughout

27. The adrenal glands

A. the right gland lies in contact with the inferior vena cava antero-medially
B. the left gland lies anterior to the pancreas
C. receive arterial branches from the renal arteries
D. the left gland is drained via one large vein which crosses the midline to drain into the inferior vena cava
E. are innervated by pre-ganglionic sympathetic fibres, the majority of which end in the medulla of the gland

28. The following statements concern the anal canal

A. the lymphatics of the lower half of the canal drain into the medial superficial inguinal lymph nodes
B. there is a portal-systemic anastomosis halfway down the canal
C. the external sphincter is innervated mainly by sympathetic fibres
D. the pubo-rectalis fibres blend with the superficial part of the external sphincter to form the ano-rectal ring
E. the lower half of the canal is lined with columnar epithelium

ANATOMY

29. The following are tributaries of the portal vein

  A. middle rectal vein
  B. ileo-colic vein
  C. right gastro-epiploic vein
  D. left gastric vein
  E. cystic vein

30. With reference to the lymphatic drainage of the breast

  A. apical axillary nodes lie in the space between the pectoralis minor and the clavicle
  B. internal thoracic lymph nodes drain the medial part of the breast
  C. some of the supraclavicular lymph nodes receive afferent lymphatics from the apical axillary nodes
  D. anterior (pectoral) axillary nodes usually lie on the pectoralis major muscle
  E. cutaneous lymphatics communicate with those of the stroma

31. The rectum

  A. is about 12" long
  B. begins at the level of the third sacral vertebra
  C. lacks peritoneal covering in its lower two thirds
  D. the upper two thirds are related anteriorly to the rectovesical pouch in the femal
  E. lies in front of the raphe of the levators ani

32. With respect to the humerus

  A. the surgical neck lies proximal to the greater and lesser tuberosities
  B. the deltoid tuberosity lies halfway down the lateral aspect of the shaft
  C. the bicipital groove accommodates the radial nerve
  D. the coronoid fossa accommodates the radial head when the elbow is flexed
  E. the lateral lip of the bicipital groove receives the insertion of pectoralis major

33. The median nerve

  A. derives its fibres from segments C6–8 and T1
  B. gives off a muscular branch to the triceps
  C. supplies the ulnar half of the flexor digitorum profundus
  D. supplies the 3rd and 4th lumbricals
  E. gives off sensory branches to the dorsal aspects of the lateral 2½ fingers

34. The radial nerve

A. derives its fibres from segments C5–8 and T1
B. gives off a muscular branch to biceps
C. gives off sensory branches to the dorsal aspects of the radial half of the hand
D. accompanies the profunda artery during its descent in the arm
E. supplies triceps

35. The following statements concern the muscles of the leg

A. plantar flexors of the foot at the ankle joint are supplied by the superficial peroneal nerve and tibial nerve
B. dorsiflexors of the foot at the ankle joint are supplied by the superficial peroneal nerve
C. all muscles of the anterior fascial compartment of the thigh are supplied by branches of the femoral nerve
D. vastus lateralis is the first part of quadriceps femoris to atrophy in knee joint disease
E. paralysis of gluteus medius and minimus seriously impairs the ability of the patient to tilt the pelvis when walking

36. The heart

A. the right atrial appendage projects to the left and overlaps the right side of the aortic root
B. the atrioventricular bundle of His passes through the central fibrous body
C. the coronary arteries are anatomical end arteries
D. the right coronary artery gives off posterior left ventricular wall arteries which appear like an inverted C on angiography
E. the sinus node artery arises from the right coronary artery in about 90% of individuals

37. The scalp

A. the pericranium is continuous with the outer layer of dura at the foramen magna
B. most of the vessels supplying the scalp lie in subcutaneous connective tissues
C. when injecting a local anaesthetic, the tip of the needle should lie in the loose areolar tissue layer deep to the galea aponeurotica
D. the emissary veins connect the dural sinuses with the veins of the scalp
E. the five layers of the scalp are intimately bound together and move as one unit

38. Considering the anatomy of the fingers

    A. the terminal branch of the digital artery passes through the pulp space
    B. the digital synovial sheaths of the index, middle and ring fingers, on the dorsal surface of the hand, are continuous with the ulnar bursa
    C. the first palmar interosseus muscle is inserted into the medial side of the base of the proximal phalanx of the thumb
    D. the flexor digitorum profundus tendons are inserted into the base of the middle phalanx
    E. the four palmar digital arteries arise mainly from the deep palmar arch

39. The skull

    A. the thinnest part of the lateral wall of the skull is where the postero-inferior part of the parietal bone articulates with the occipital bone
    B. the pterion overlies the anterior division of the middle meningeal artery and vein
    C. fractures of the mandible most commonly occur at the ramus
    D. the VIIth and VIIIth cranial nerves pass through the petrous part of the temporal bone
    E. the inner table of the skull bones is thinner and more brittle than the outer table

40. The following muscles and nerves supplying them are correctly linked

    A. chief supinator of the forearm – deep branch of the radial nerve
    B. extensors of the hand at the wrist joint – deep branch of the radial nerve
    C. all muscles of the anterior fascial compartment of the forearm – median nerve
    D. palmar and dorsal interossei – deep branch of the ulnar nerve
    E. 3rd and 4th lumbricals – median nerve

41. The following cutaneous areas and supplying sensory roots are correctly paired

    A. the sole of the foot – S3
    B. the little finger – T1
    C. the groin – L5
    D. the umbilicus – T10
    E. the index finger – C5

42. The following nerves and plexus roots are correctly paired

- A. femoral nerve – L2, 3, 4
- B. ilioinguinal nerve – L2
- C. obturator nerve – S2, 3, 4
- D. iliohypogastric nerve – T12, L1
- E. genito-femoral nerve – L3, 4

43. The following structures lie behind the left kidney

- A. 12th rib
- B. tail of pancreas
- C. left ilio-inguinal nerve
- D. spleen
- E. left lung

44. The kidneys

- A. have segmental blood supply
- B. have the same nerve supply as the large intestine
- C. are separated from the 12th rib by the pleura and the diaphragm
- D. renal arteries arise from the abdominal aorta at the level of L4 vertebra
- E. are crossed anteriorly by the iliohypogastric and ilionguinal nerves

45. The structure of the skin

- A. the deep cutaneous vascular (reticular) plexus lies at the junction of the reticular and papillary layers of the dermis
- B. Langerhans cells have receptors for the Fc portion of IgG
- C. collagen fibres of the reticular dermis are mainly type III
- D. surgical incisions perpendicular to Kriessl's lines minimize post-operative scarring
- E. in the predominant pattern of blood supply to the skin, vessels from the aorta or its major branches form direct cutaneous arteries which lie superficial to the muscles and parallel to the skin for long distances

46. The statements below concern skin grafts and flaps which are eventually re-anastomosed

- A. split thickness grafts contain all the dermis
- B. full thickness grafts have a vascular pedicle which is re-anastomosed in a recipient site
- C. bare cortical bone is an acceptable recipient site for a full thickness graft
- D. hair growth and sweating are fairly well preserved in skin flaps
- E. all skin flaps have a vascular 'pedicle' which is re-anastomosed in a recipient site

ANATOMY

47. Considering the normal histology of the stomach

    A.   parietal cells are found mainly in the upper half of the gastric glands
    B.   the number of tubovesicles in resting parietal cells increases when these cells are stimulated to produce HCl
    C.   parietal cells release one HCO_3^- to accompany every H^+ secreted into the lumen
    D.   chief cells produce intrinsic factor
    E.   argentaffin cells are not confined to the stomach but are found throughout the digestive tract

48. During Syme's operation (amputation in the region of the ankle), the surgeon will encounter the following structures lying behind and below the medial malleolus

    A.   extensor hallucis longus
    B.   posterior tibial nerve
    C.   flexor digitorum longus
    D.   peroneus tertius
    E.   tibialis posterior

49. Injury to the medial cord of the brachial plexus results in

    A.   paralysis of all the intrinsic muscles of the hand
    B.   loss of elbow flexion
    C.   loss of cutaneous sensations over the anterior surface of palm and fingers
    D.   paralysis of the long flexors of the fingers
    E.   paralysis of the pronator teres

50. The following muscles assist in the inversion of the foot

    A.   tibialis anterior
    B.   tibialis posterior
    C.   peroneus longus
    D.   all tendons of extensor digitorum longus
    E.   flexor hallucis longus

51. With respect to intravenous excretory urography

    A.   the contrast media used are water soluble
    B.   the nephrographic phase is seen in films taken 20 minutes after injecting the contrast medium
    C.   the pyelographic phase can be enhanced by tilting the patient into the Trendelenburg position
    D.   the post-micturition cystogram is an accurate means of measuring the amount of residual urine
    E.   the ureters are seen to lie on the tips of the transverse processes of the lumbar vertebrae

52. The following statements concern the blood supply of the small and large intestine

A. the upper half of the duodenum is supplied by the inferior pancreatico-duodenal artery, a branch of the superior mesenteric artery
B. the jejunum and ileum are supplied by branches of the superior mesenteric artery
C. the ascending colon is supplied by the middle colic artery
D. the distal third of the transverse colon is supplied by the superior left colic artery, a branch of the inferior mesenteric artery
E. the descending colon is supplied by the superior and inferior left colic arteries, branches of the inferior mesenteric artery

53. The histological features of a normal node include

A. specialized postcapillary venules in the paracortex
B. abundance of B lymphocytes in the paracortical zone
C. Reed–Sternberg cells
D. macrophages adherent to sinus endothelia
E. Congo red staining with green birefringence in polarized light

54. Considering the anatomy of the kidney and the ureter

A. the left kidney is related to the pancreas anteriorly
B. segmental (terminal) branches of the renal artery exhibit excellent anastomoses with one another
C. accessory renal arteries, when present, usually arise from the abdominal aorta
D. the perirenal capsule (Gerota's fascia) encloses the kidney and the adrenal gland together
E. the ureter crosses anterior to the genitofemoral nerve

55. The paranasal sinuses

A. the ethmoidal sinuses are separated from the orbit by a thin plate of bone
B. the hiatus semilunaris lie low down on the medial wall of the sinus
C. the frontal and posterior ethmoidal sinuses drain into the infundibulum
D. the infundibulum drains into the hiatus semilunaris (the maxillary opening)
E. the mucous membrane of the sphenoidal sinuses is supplied by the posterior ethmoidal nerves

ANATOMY

56. With reference to the hip joint

- A. the subpsoas bursa communicates with the hip joint in most cases
- B. rectus femoris frequently has a sesamoid bone which lies just below the anterior inferior iliac spine
- C. the iliofemoral ligament is attached to anterior superior iliac spine
- D. gluteus medius passes lateral to the joint capsule to be inserted into the lesser trochanter
- E. traumatic posterior dislocation of the joint occurs more commonly than anterior dislocation

57. Consider the following postero-anterior plain film of the chest (Figure 1)

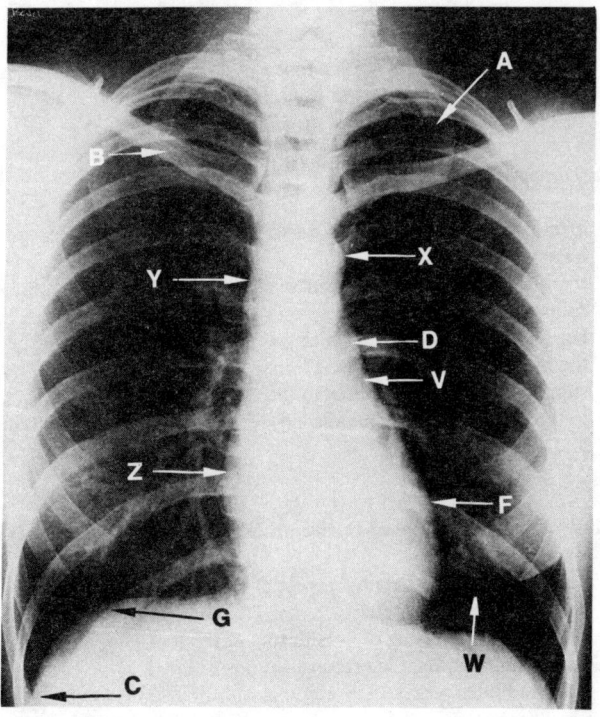

Figure 1

The following statements are correct

- A. 'X' is the aortic knuckle
- B. 'Y' is the border of the right auricle
- C. 'Z' is the right ventricle
- D. 'W' is a breast shadow
- E. 'V' is the left auricle

58. The brachial plexus

A. is formed by the junction of the anterior rami of C1–8
B. the divisions of the plexus lie on the serratus anterior and subscapularis muscles
C. the cords of the plexus lie within the longus colli muscle in the neck
D. the radial nerve represents a continuation of the posterior cord
E. the superior trunk of the plexus is the trunk which is usually involved in the thoracic outlet syndrome

59. The clinical features of an injury to the common peroneal nerve due to a fracture of the neck of the fibula include

A. paralysis of tibialis anterior
B. positive Trendelenburg test
C. paralysis of peroneus longus
D. equinovarus deformity of the foot
E. calcaneovalgus deformity of the foot

60. The facial nerve

A. gives off the chorda tympani nerve 5 mm below the stylomastoid foramen
B. if injured along its vertical course within the mastoid bone, the stapedius reflex would be normal
C. has a mandibular branch which passes about 2.5 cm behind the angle of the mandible
D. supplies secretomotor fibres to the submandibular gland
E. in the bony wall of the middle ear, lies posterior to the mastoid antrum and air cells

61. The clinical features of a lumbar disc prolapse affecting root S1 only include

A. paraesthesia on the medial aspect of the foot
B. a positive femoral stretch
C. weakness and wasting of dorsiflexors of the foot
D. limitation of straight leg raising
E. impaired knee jerk

62. When performing a highly selective vagotomy for duodenal ulcer, the surgeon usually

A. finds that the anterior vagus gives off branches to the liver and gallbladder
B. finds the posterior vagus as a thick cord closely applied to the oesophagus
C. denervates the parietal area of the stomach
D. divides the coeliac branch of the posterior vagus
E. performs pyloroplasty

ANATOMY

63. Consider the CT scan of the abdomen (post-contrast film) (Figure 2)

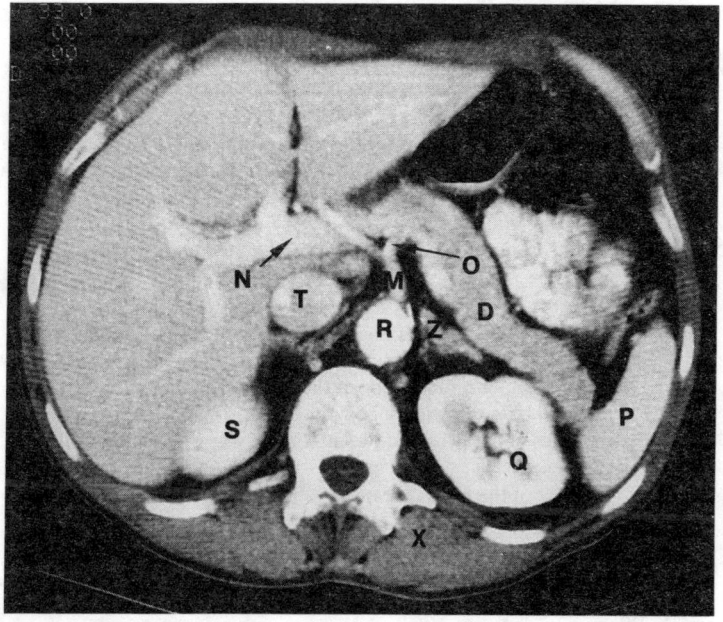

Figure 2

The following statements are correct

- A. 'N' is the main portal vein
- B. 'M' is the common bile duct
- C. 'P' is the left kidney
- D. 'T' is the inferior vena cava
- E. this cut lies at the level of the second lumbar vertebra

64. The testis and scrotum

- A. lymphatic drainage of the testis takes place to para-aortic lymph nodes at the level of L4
- B. when tapping a hydrocele, the cannula traverses the visceral layer of tunica vaginalis
- C. lymphatic drainage of the scrotum takes place to the medial group of superficial lymph nodes
- D. the epididymis is attached to the posterior border of the testis
- E. right and left testicular veins drain directly into the inferior vena cava

65. The oesophagus

A. the lymphatic drainage of the lower third ends in the coeliac lymph nodes
B. in the lower third oesophageal tributaries of the azygos veins anastomose with tributaries of the left gastro-epiploic vein
C. the left recurrent laryngeal nerve lies posterior to the thoracic part of the oesophagus
D. the left bronchus constricts the oesophagus as it crosses anterior to it
E. the lower third is the commonest site for carcinoma of the oesophagus

66. The following statements concern the prostate and male urethra

A. the prostatic urethra is the narrowest part of the urethra
B. the membranous urethra is surrounded by fibres of the external sphincter
C. the median, or middle, lobe of the prostate contain more glandular material than the other lobes
D. the veins of the prostatic venous plexus, which have thin walls, are valveless
E. all lobes of the prostate can be palpated through the rectum

67. The histological features of a transverse section through a normal appendix include

A. crypts of Leiberkühn
B. avascular submucosa
C. lymphatic follicles with germ centres in the lamina propria
D. muscularis externa consisting of outer circular and inner longitudinal layers of smooth muscle
E. fibrinopurulent exudate on the surface

68. The histology of a normal parotid gland usually shows

A. a well-developed capsule with septa subdividing the gland into lobes and lobules
B. striated ducts whose columnar cells have their nuclei located at the base of the cell
C. squamous epithelium in a mucoid stroma
D. cribriform nests of cells separated by strands of hyalinized connective tissue
E. serous alveoli

69. The peritoneum

A. peritoneal fluid contains leukocytes and antibodies
B. the nerve supply to the centre of the diaphragmatic peritoneum has the same segmental origin as the lower six thoracic nerves
C. the free border of the lesser omentum lies anterior to the epiploic foramen
D. the parietal peritoneum is devoid of sensory nerves
E. the peritoneum is a semipermeable membrane

70. The following differences help the operating surgeon to distinguish between jejunum and ileum

A. the calibre of the small bowel diminishes from proximal jejunum to distal ileum
B. Peyer's patches are more numerous in the ileum than in the jejunum
C. the ileal mesentery is thinner and more translucent than that of the jejunum
D. there is a more marked tendency towards arborization and anastomosis of vascular archades in the jejunal mesentery than in that of the ileum
E. the lymphatics and lymph nodes are more numerous and larger in the ileal mesentery than in that of the jejunum

71. With respect to the gallbladder and common bile duct (CBD)

A. the cystic artery branches from the right hepatic artery and lies most commonly between the cystic duct and liver
B. the right hepatic duct rarely enters the gallbladder near its junction with the cystic duct
C. the internal diameter of a normal CBD is about 12 mm on ultrasonography
D. the wall of the supraduodenal part of the CBD has a venous plexus which can be seen at operation
E. when performing cholecystectomy through Kocher's incision the surgeon must not divide the rectus muscle

72. In the root of the neck

A. the subclavian vein crosses the first rib posterior to scalenus anterior
B. the phrenic nerve descends anterior to scalenus anterior
C. the cervical dome of pleura lies behind scalenus medius
D. the stellate ganglion lies at the level of C7 vertebra
E. the subclavian artery crosses the first rib anterior to scalenus anterior

73. The greater omentum

A. is a four-layered serous structure
B. acts as a plug in acute abdominal inflammation
C. occasionally has congenital openings
D. is mainly supplied by the left gastric artery
E. lies posterior to the transverse colon

74. The spinal cord

A. the subdural space contains the cerebrospinal fluid (CSF)
B. the cord segment T12 lies at the level of vertebral body T11
C. two-point discrimination sense travels in the lateral white column
D. hemisection of the cord results in contralateral upper motor neuron paralysis below the level of the lesion
E. hemisection of the cord results in contralateral loss of pain and temperature sense below the lesion

75. The rectum

A. possesses appendices epiploicae
B. has peritoneal covering throughout its length
C. exhibits three lateral curves, two with their convexities toward the left and one with its convexity toward the right
D. Denoviller's fascia, which is the line of separation between the anorectal and urogenital pelvises, is more developed in the female than in the male
E. the middle and inferior rectal arteries are branches of the inferior mesenteric artery

76. Sternocleidomastoid muscle

A. arises from a medial sternal head and a lateral clavicular head
B. is primarily supplied by branches from the brachial plexus
C. has a thick venous plexus deep to the anterior sheath
D. when both muscles work in unison, they extend the neck posteriorly
E. the cervical sympathetic chain and ganglia lie deep to the muscle

77. The adrenal glands

A. are retroperitoneal organs
B. the left suprarenal vein usually joins the left inferior phrenic vein
C. are purely mesodermal in origin
D. efferent lymphatics drain into the highest lumbar nodes
E. the left gland is usually more difficult to explore and remove surgically than the right gland

ANATOMY

78. Porto-systemic anastomoses occur in the following sites

    A.   around the umbilicus
    B.   the middle third of the oesophagus
    C.   the lower end of the rectum
    D.   the bare area of the liver
    E.   the appendix

79. In the femoral triangle

    A.   sartorius muscle forms the medial border
    B.   the lateral circumflex vein frequently crosses profunda femoris just distal to its origin
    C.   the common femoral artery gives off the deep circumflex iliac artery
    D.   profunda femoris artery arises from the medial aspect of the common femoral artery
    E.   the femoral vein lies medial to the femoral canal

80. The following structures are found in the subplatysmal space (deep to the platysma and superficial to the deep cervical fascia)

    A.   the mandibular branch of the facial nerve
    B.   the submental venous plexus
    C.   the carotid sheath
    D.   the descending cervical branch of the facial nerve
    E.   sternocleidomastoid muscle

81. Intercostal structures

    A.   transversus thoracis muscle lies between the external and internal intercostal muscles
    B.   intercostal neurovascular structures pass behind the superior border of the corresponding rib
    C.   anterior intercostal arteries of the first five spaces come off the thoracic aorta
    D.   intercostal arteries and nerves lie superficial to the transversus thoracis
    E.   the first intercostal nerve gives off an anterior cutaneous branch

82. The pharynx

    A.   the palatine tonsils drain into the deep cervical lymph nodes
    B.   the potential gap between the middle and lower fibres of the superior constrictor muscle is the usual site of the pharyngeal pouch
    C.   the pharyngeal mucous membrane is continuous with that of the tympanic cavity
    D.   the piriform fossa is bounded laterally by the aryepiglottic folds
    E.   the nasopharyngeal tonsils are smallest in childhood and reach their maximum size after puberty

83. The ulnar nerve supplies the following muscles in the hand

   A.   adductor pollicis
   B.   all dorsal interossei
   C.   the lateral two lumbricals
   D.   abductor pollicis brevis
   E.   all hypothenar muscles

84. With respect to the spleen

   A.   the splenic artery passes to the spleen through the gastrosplenic ligament
   B.   the lienorenal ligament contains the tail of the pancreas
   C.   most laterally, the spleen is in contact with the phrenico-colic ligament
   D.   segmental resection of the spleen is possible due to segmental blood supply
   E.   splenectomy may be performed through a left subcostal incision

85. With respect to the neck region

   A.   the submandibular gland comes into direct contact with the sublingual glands
   B.   branchial cleft cysts usually lie superficial to sternocleidomastoid
   C.   some of the submandibular lymph nodes lie within the submandibular salivary gland
   D.   the mylohyoid cleft connects the neck to the oral cavity
   E.   the thyroid isthmus usually lies at the level of the upper three tracheal rings

86. The anterior abdominal wall

   A.   the dermatome over the umbilicus corresponds to root T12
   B.   the skin, above the level of the umbilicus, drains into the anterior axillary lymph nodes
   C.   the lateral thoracic vein anastomoses with the superficial epigastric vein
   D.   the potential space beneath Scarpa's fascia opens into the thigh
   E.   the presence of a patent urachus may result in an umbilical fecal fistula

87. Consider the following schematic coronal section of part of the pelvis and perineum (Figure 3)

   The following statements are true:
   A.   'X' represents the internal anal sphincter
   B.   the muscular structure 'Y' represents the levators ani
   C.   internal haemorrhoids usually develop below the pectinate line
   D.   the anal glands frequently penetrate the internal sphincter to end in the intersphincteric plane
   E.   the lymphatic drainage of the mucosa below the pectinate line is similar to that of the rectum

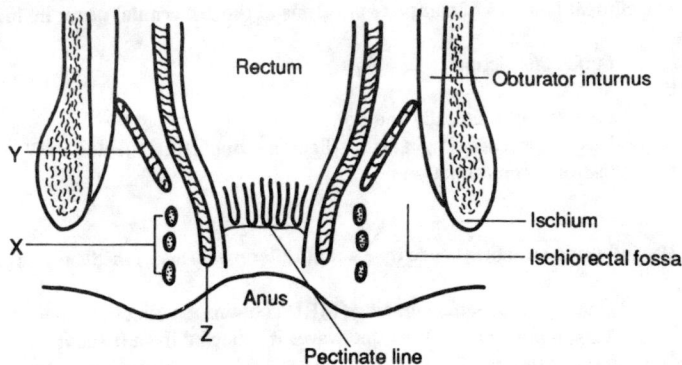

Figure 3

88. With respect to the pituitary gland

  A. the posterior lobe develops from Rathke's pouch
  B. the posterior lobe synthesizes ADH
  C. the optic chiasma is separated from the anterior lobe by the diaphragma sella
  D. in trans-sphenoidal hypophysectomy the floor of the sella turcica is removed
  E. the oculomotor nerve passes in the medial wall of the cavernous sinus lateral to the gland

89. The parotid gland

  A. the facial nerve lies between the superficial and the deep parts of the gland
  B. the parotid duct passes forward deep to the masseter muscle
  C. the gland is enclosed in a dense fibrous capsule
  D. parasympathetic secretomotor fibres reach the parotid via the great auricular nerve
  E. the glenoid process extends medially behind the temporomandibular joint

90. The long saphenous vein usually receives the following tributaries in the femoral triangle

  A. the superficial epigastric vein
  B. the deep circumflex iliac vein
  C. the deep external pudendal vein
  D. the lateral accessory vein
  E. the superficial circumflex iliac vein

91. The clinical features of complete paralysis of the 3rd cranial nerve include

- A. pupil constriction
- B. ptosis
- C. the eye looks laterally and downward
- D. loss of consensual light reflex (light is shone in the affected eye)
- E. loss of accommodation reflex

92. The following statements are true about different forms of medical imaging

- A. magnetic resonance imaging (MRI) contains ionizing radiation
- B. a small portion of ultrasound waves is reflected from tissue interfaces back to the transducer
- C. no ill-effects of ultrasound scanning have been discovered when used at diagnostic intensity levels
- D. computerized tomography (CT) shows small differences in tissue density between the grey matter and the white matter of the brain
- E. in CT imaging atomic nuclei within an area of the patient's body align in a strong magnetic field

93. In laparotomy incisions

- A. rectus abdominis must be divided in a paramedian incision
- B. the risk of damaging the nerve supply to the rectus, in a paramedian incision, can be minimized by making the incision as lateral as possible
- C. it is more important to suture the external oblique fascia than the linear alba when suturing a lower midline incision
- D. drainage tubes should be inserted through the main incision
- E. the 9th intercostal nerve is encountered in Kocher's incision

94. The tonsil (palatine)

- A. lies in direct contact with the medial surface of the superior constrictor muscle of the pharynx
- B. is separated from the glossopharyngeal nerve by the superior constrictor muscle
- C. has a thin fibrous capsule which is continuous with the pharyngeal aponeurosis
- D. may contain bone
- E. is partly supplied by the inferior tonsillar artery which branches from the descending palatine artery

95. With reference to development of the gastro-intestinal tract

- A. the primitive intestinal loop normally rotates 90° in a clockwise direction
- B. when the primitive intestinal loop rotates 90° counterclockwise, the colon and caecum settle in the left side of the abdominal cavity
- C. duodenal atresia is thought to result from incomplete recanalization of the lumen
- D. the rectum is the commonest site for duplications of the gastro-intestinal tract
- E. gastroschisis is usually associated with exstrophy of the urinary bladder

96. Considering the development of the gastro-intestinal tract

- A. the pectinate line forms the junction between endodermal and ectodermal parts of the anal canal
- B. congenital umbilical hernia results when intestinal loops fail to return to the abdominal cavity around the end of the third month
- C. muscular layers and skin around the umbilicus are absent in congenital umbilical hernia
- D. Meckel's diverticulum may contain gastric mucosa
- E. vitelline ligaments predispose to intestinal volvulus

97. The following statements concern the development of the urogenital system

- A. connection failure between excretory and collecting systems may result in congenital polycystic kidneys
- B. duplication of the ureter usually results from early splitting of the metanephric blastema
- C. hypospadias results from incomplete fusion of the urethral folds
- D. the testis normally travels through the inguinal canal during the third month of development
- E. horseshoe kidney affects about 1 in 600 people

98. The palatine tonsil

- A. is separated from the superior constrictor muscle by lax connective tissue
- B. receives blood supply from the facial artery
- C. lies anterior to the palatoglossal arch
- D. is separated from the glossopharyngeal nerve by the superior constrictor muscle of the pharynx
- E. receives blood supply from the ascending pharyngeal artery

99. In development of the heart

- A. anterior displacement of the trunco-conal septum results in Fallot's tetralogy
- B. incomplete fusion of the trunco-conal ridges usually results in transposition of the great vessels
- C. tricuspid atresia is nearly always associated with ventricular septal defect
- D. premature closure of the foramen ovale results in underdevelopment of the right ventricle
- E. ostium secundum may arise from excessive resorption of the septum primum

100. With respect to development of the thyroid gland

- A. follicular cells arise from the epithelium of the dorsal wing of the fourth pharyngeal pouch
- B. parafollicular cells arise from the fifth pharyngeal pouch
- C. approximately 50% of thyroglossal cysts lie close to or just inferior to the body of the hyoid bone
- D. thyroglossal cysts may lie at the base of the tongue
- E. a thyroglossal fistula usually arises due to rupture of a thyroglossal cyst

Answers

1.
 - A. (F) the external oblique fibres run parallel to the skin incision
 - B. (T)
 - C. (F) Scarpa's fascia is superficial to the external oblique
 - D. (T)
 - E. (F) the appendicular artery has no anastomosis. This explains the vulnerability of the appendix to necrosis and perforation once the artery is blocked

2.
 - A. (F) passes in front of the medial malleolus
 - B. (T)
 - C. (F) usually in front of this artery, but it may lie behind it
 - D. (F) it has more numerous tributaries at this level, and this fact helps to distinguish it from the femoral vein during surgery
 - E. (T)

3.
 - A. (F) the ethmoidal and sphenoidal air sinuses produce a composite shadow
 - B. (T)
 - C. (F) the film cassette is positioned against the nose and forehead
 - D. (T)
 - E. (T)

4.
A.	(F)	the popliteal artery is the deepest structure in the popliteal fossa
B.	(T)	
C.	(T)	
D.	(F)	this is part of the medial boundary of the popliteal fossa
E.	(T)	

NB. The popliteal artery is usually exposed through a medial approach when performing a femoropopliteal or ileopopliteal bypass (Figure 4)

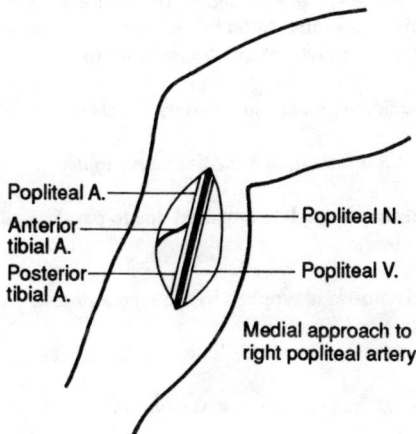

Figure 4

5.
A.	(F)	passes behind the fossa
B.	(F)	this is confirmed in kidney transplantation
C.	(T)	therefore the surgeon should divide the medial fascia when mobilizing the left ureter
D.	(F)	the uterine artery crosses anterior to it
E.	(T)	

6.
A.	(F)	on the superior surface
B.	(T)	
C.	(F)	to iliac nodes. Only a small amount of pelvic lymph reaches the inguinal nodes
D.	(F)	on the pelvic surface of the piriformis muscles
E.	(T)	

7.
A.	(F)	the angle is about 125° in the adult, but it is larger in the young child
B.	(F)	the intertrochanteric line connects them anteriorly, and the intertrochanteric crest connects them posteriorly
C.	(T)	
D.	(F)	the fibres are attached to the lesser trochanter
E.	(T)	

8.
A.	(F)	this branch reaches the head along the ligament of the head
B.	(F)	it is less important than the other two routes of blood supply: the retinacular vessels travelling in the posterior capsule and the medullary vessels in the femoral neck
C.	(T)	
D.	(F)	
E.	(T)	the small blood supply through the ligamentum teres is insufficient to maintain the head viable

9.
A.	(F)	this results from damage to the common peroneal nerve
B.	(F)	this area is innervated by the common peroneal nerve
C.	(T)	due to paralysis of quadriceps femoris
D.	(T)	
E.	(F)	the adductors are supplied by the obturator nerve

10.
A.	(F)	this is a feature of a median nerve injury
B.	(T)	
C.	(F)	this is only slightly impaired due to paralysis of the adductor pollicis
D.	(T)	
E.	(F)	this muscle is supplied by the median nerve

11.
A.	(F)	it normally lies on the line
B.	(T)	
C.	(F)	lies at the level of the lower border of T4
D.	(T)	
E.	(T)	

12.
A.	(T)	the posterior half is firmly attached to deep and oblique portions of the tibial collateral ligament
B.	(F)	to the deep and oblique portions
C.	(T)	
D.	(T)	
E.	(F)	the central part is avascular. This implies that only peripheral lesions can be repaired

13.
A.	(F)	posterior to it
B.	(T)	
C.	(F)	usually from the right hepatic artery
D.	(T)	
E.	(T)	

14.
A.	(F)	it bulges medial to the artery
B.	(T)	
C.	(F)	the indirect hernia is the commonest hernia
D.	(T)	due to weaker abdominal muscles
E.	(T)	due to the narrow orifice at the internal ring

15.
A.	(T)	
B.	(T)	

ANATOMY

	C.	(T)	
	D.	(F)	the genital branch of the genito-femoral nerve is part of it
	E.	(T)	

16.
A.	(F)	by the fascia transversalis
B.	(T)	
C.	(F)	it transmits the ilio-inguinal nerve
D.	(T)	the deep ring moves laterally as a result of growth
E.	(T)	

17.
A.	(T)	
B.	(F)	it is formed by the lowest arching fibres of the internal oblique and transversus abdominis
C.	(F)	this re-inforcement lies in the medial third
D.	(T)	
E.	(F)	it lies lateral to these vessels

18.
A.	(T)	this nerve may be damaged in shoulder dislocation
B.	(T)	
C.	(T)	anterior dislocation is much commoner accounting for about 97% of cases
D.	(F)	the abduction angle is decreased. This is seen in patients who had surgery for recurrent dislocation whereby the subscapularis muscle is shortened preventing external rotation
E.	(F)	the anterior approach is usually used in arthroplasty

19.
A.	(T)	
B.	(T)	
C.	(F)	
D.	(T)	
E.	(T)	

20.
A.	(F)	from the first part
B.	(F)	this is true of the vertebral artery
C.	(T)	
D.	(F)	this is a branch of the costocervical trunk
E.	(F)	this is a branch of the costocervical trunk

21.
A.	(T)	
B.	(T)	
C.	(F)	deep to it
D.	(T)	
E.	(F)	deep to it

22.
A.	(F)	
B.	(T)	
C.	(T)	this is the first vessel to be encountered in thyroidectomy
D.	(T)	care should be taken not to remove the parathyroid glands during thyroidectomy
E.	(F)	the external laryngeal nerve is closely related to the superior thyroid artery, whereas the recurrent laryngeal nerve may be closely related to the inferior thyroid artery

23.
- A. (T)
- B. (T) this causes shoulder drop
- C. (T) because the deep cervical lymph nodes are closely attached to it
- D. (F)
- E. (F)

24.
- A. (F) this is a branch of the external carotid
- B. (T)
- C. (T)
- D. (T)
- E. (F) the two inferior thyroid veins anastomose and drain into the left brachio-cephalic veins

25.
- A. (F) parasympathetic innervation (S3–S4)
- B. (T)
- C. (T)
- D. (F) spinal nerves (S2–S3)
- E. (T)

See Figure 4a

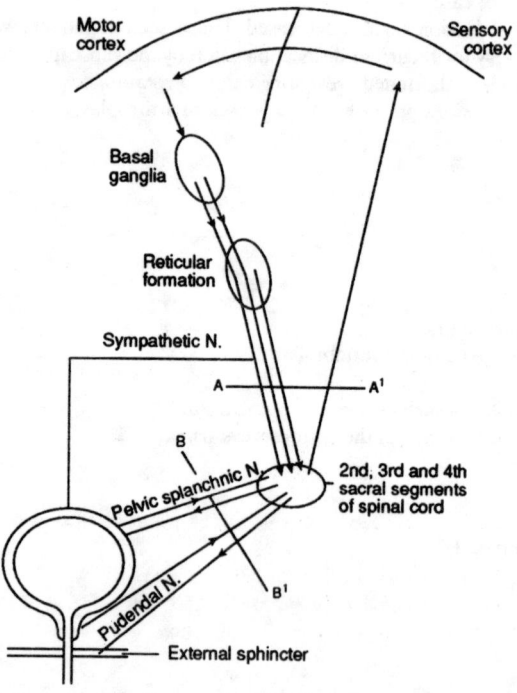

Figure 4a. The innervation of the bladder

26.
- A. (F) below the 2nd arch and above the 3rd
- B. (T) the fistula passes between the structures of the 2nd and 3rd arches
- C. (T)
- D. (T) 'complete fistula'
- E. (F) the lateral part is lined with squamous epithelium and the medial part with ciliated columnar epithelium

27.
- A. (T)
- B. (F) it lies behind the pancreas
- C. (T)
- D. (F) it drains into either the left renal vein or the left inferior phrenic vein
- E. (T)

28.
- A. (T) enlargement of such nodes may be the presentation of anal carcinoma
- B. (T) the superior rectal vein drains into the portal system whereas the middle and inferior rectal veins drain into the systemic circulation
- C. (F) the external sphincter is made of striped muscle and is innervated by the inferior rectal nerve branch of the pudendal nerve
- D. (F) the pubo-rectalis fibres blend with the deep part of the external sphincter and with the internal sphincter to form the ano-rectal ring
- E. (F) it is lined with stratified squamous epithelium

29.
- A. (F) this drains into the internal iliac vein
- B. (T)
- C. (T)
- D. (T)
- E. (T)

30.
- A. (T)
- B. (T)
- C. (T) the nodes in the lower part of the posterior triangle
- D. (F) these nodes lie under cover of the muscle
- E. (T)

31.
- A. (F) when it is straightened out, it measures about 5" in length
- B. (T)
- C. (F) it is devoid of peritoneal covering in its lower third
- D. (F) this is true in the male. In the female the recto-uterine pouch with its contents lies in front of the rectum
- E. (T)

32.
- A. (F) the surgical neck lies distal to the tuberosities, whereas the anatomical neck lies immediately below the head
- B. (T)
- C. (F) the spiral groove behind and below the deltoid tuberosity

			accommodates this nerve
	D.	(F)	it accommodates the coronoid process of the ulna, during elbow flexion
	E.	(T)	

33.
	A.	(T)	
	B.	(F)	it gives off no branches in the arm
	C.	(F)	this is supplied by the ulnar nerve
	D.	(F)	it supplies the first two lumbricals
	E.	(F)	it innervates the palmar aspects of the lateral 3½ fingers

34.
	A.	(T)	
	B.	(F)	the biceps is supplied by the musculocutaneous nerve
	C.	(T)	
	D.	(T)	
	E.	(T)	

35.
	A.	(T)	
	B.	(F)	the deep peroneal nerve
	C.	(F)	psoas is supplied by branches from the lumbar plexus. The femoral nerve supplies the others (quadriceps femoris, pectineus, iliacus and sartorius)
	D.	(F)	vastus medialis is the first part to atrophy in knee joint disease and last to recover
	E.	(T)	

36.
	A.	(T)	the angiographic appearance of the atrial appendages helps to distinguish between the left and right atrium
	B.	(T)	in this position it lies close to the mitral, aortic and tricuspid valves
	C.	(F)	there are some anastomoses between the two coronaries, e.g. Vieussens' ring, Kugel's artery and between the anterior and posterior descending arteries. It should be noted that these anastomoses may not be sufficient to prevent an infarction once an artery has been blocked
	D.	(T)	
	E.	(F)	only in about 55% of cases. In the remaining 45% of cases it arises from the circumflex artery

37.
	A.	(T)	
	B.	(T)	
	C.	(F)	the nerves supplying the scalp lie mainly in the subcutaneous connective tissue which lies superficial to galea aponeurotica
	D.	(T)	these valveless veins traverse the loose areolar tissue
	E.	(F)	the skin, subcutaneous connective tissue and galea aponeurotica are intimately bound together

38.
	A.	(T)	this explains how necrosis of the diaphyses of the distal phalanx may complicate pulp space infection which can cause thrombosis of this artery

ANATOMY

- B. (F) these sheaths commence at the level of the distal transverse crease of the palm
- C. (T)
- D. (F) each tendon of the FDP passes through a division in the FDS tendon then continues downward to its insertion into the base of the distal phalanx
- E. (F) from the superficial palmar arch

39.
- A. (F) the thinnest part is the pterion which is located where the antero-inferior corner of the parietal bone articulates with the greater wing of the sphenoid
- B. (T) injury at this site may result in extradural haemorrhage
- C. (F) the neck of the mandible is the commonest site
- D. (T)
- E. (T)

40.
- A. (F) biceps brachialis is the chief supinator. It is innervated by the musculo-cutaneous nerve
- B. (T)
- C. (F) the ulnar nerve supplies flexor carpi ulnaris and the medial part of flexor digitorum profundus
- D. (T)
- E. (F) 1st and 2nd lumbricals are supplied by the median nerve. 3rd and 4th lumbricals are supplied by the deep branch of the ulnar nerve

41.
- A. (F) S1
- B. (T)
- C. (F) L1
- D. (T)
- E. (F) C7

42.
- A. (T)
- B. (F) L1
- C. (F) L2, 3, 4
- D. (T)
- E. (F) L1, 2

43.
- A. (T)
- B. (F) in front of the left kidney
- C. (T) traversing quadratus lumborum
- D. (F) in front of the left kidney
- E. (T)

44.
- A. (T) this makes segmental resection possible. It also defines an avascular plane for nephrolithotomy
- B. (T) T10, T11 and T12 through the lesser and lowest splanchnic nerves. Hence acute large bowel obstruction may occur in renal colic
- C. (T)
- D. (F) at the level of L1/L2 intervertebral disc
- E. (F) these lie posterior to the kidneys

45.
- A. (F) the deep plexus lies at the interface between the reticular layer and the superficial fascia
- B. (T) they are immunologically active (graft rejection)
- C. (F) they are mainly type I except in early development when type III predominate
- D. (F) incisions parallel to these cleavage lines minimize scarring
- E. (F) in the predominant pattern, the main segmental artery lies deep to the muscle. This gives perforating branches through the muscles (musculocutaneous arteries)

46.
- A. (F) contain part of the dermis
- B. (F) this is true of skin flaps
- C. (F) unacceptable as it is unable to provide vascularity to the graft
- D. (T)
- E. (T)

47.
- A. (T)
- B. (F) the number of tubovesicles decreases as these structures fuse with the plasmalemma to form microvilli
- C. (F) for every H^+ secreted into the gastric lumen, one HCO_3^- is released into the blood
- D. (F) intrinsic factor is produced by parietal cells. Chief cells are zymogenic, i.e. produce pepsin and lipase
- E. (T) carcinoid tumours are derived from these cells

48.
- A. (F)
- B. (T)
- C. (T)
- D. (F)
- E. (T)

A and D lie anterior to the ankle joint

49.
- A. (T)
- B. (F)
- C. (T)
- D. (T)
- E. (F) supplied by the lateral head of the median nerve

NB. The medial cord branches include: 1) the medial head of the median nerve; 2) the ulnar nerve; 3) the medial pectoral nerve; 4) the medial cutaneous nerve of the arm; 5) the medial cutaneous nerve of the forearm

50.
- A. (T)
- B. (T)
- C. (F) it is an everter
- D. (F) only the medial tendons assist in inversion, whereas the lateral tendons assist in eversion
- E. (F) this muscle assists in plantar flexion

51.
A.	(T)	
B.	(F)	the nephrogram is seen immediately after finishing the injection
C.	(T)	
D.	(F)	it is not reliable for this purpose. However, it may reveal filling defects or the size of diverticulae
E.	(T)	

52.
A.	(F)	it is supplied by the superior pancreatico-duodenal artery, a branch of the gastro-duodenal artery
B.	(T)	these branches lie between the two layers of the mesentery
C.	(F)	it is supplied by the ileo-colic and right colic arteries
D.	(T)	
E.	(T)	

53.
A.	(T)	these are functionally important
B.	(F)	T-lymphocytes predominate in this zone
C.	(F)	this is diagnostic of Hodgkin's lymphoma
D.	(T)	
E.	(F)	this is diagnostic of amyloidosis

54.
A.	(T)	
B.	(F)	there is very little communication between these branches. This explains why segmental infarction follows occlusion of these vessels
C.	(T)	when these arteries run to the lower renal pole, they may compress the ureter resulting in hydronephrosis
D.	(F)	the adrenal gland is not included. Therefore Gerota's space can be entered to remove the kidney without injuring the adrenal gland
E.	(T)	this may explain the distribution of referred pain seen in ureteral disease

55.
A.	(T)	therefore infection may readily spread to the orbit
B.	(F)	unfortunately it lies high up. Therefore fluid tends to accumulate in the sinus
C.	(F)	the frontal and anterior ethmoidal sinuses drain into the infundibulum
D.	(T)	this allows infection to spead from the anterior ethmoidal and frontal sinuses into the maxillary sinuses
E.	(T)	

56.
A.	(F)	only in about 10% of cases
B.	(T)	this may be mistaken for a fracture on plain radiographs
C.	(F)	to the anterior inferior iliac spine
D.	(F)	into the greater trochanter
E.	(T)	about 80% of dislocations are posterior

57.
A.	(T)	produced by the aortic arch
B.	(F)	'Y' represents the superior vena cava
C.	(F)	'Z' is part of the right atrium

D. (T) the subject is female
E. (T)

Also: 'A' represents the 1st rib (left); 'B' the right clavicle; 'C' the right costo-phrenic angle; 'D' the left pulmonary artery; 'F' the left ventricle; 'G' the left dome of diaphragm under which the dense liver lies

58.
A. (F) rami C5–8 with part of T1
B. (T) six divisions
C. (F) the cords are formed at the level of the first rib
D. (T)
E. (F) the inferior trunk C8–T1 is usually involved in the thoracic outlet syndrome

59.
A. (T)
B. (F)
C. (T)
D. (T) the foot is plantar-flexed and inverted
E. (F) this results from injuries to the tibial nerve. It is the opposite of equinovarus

60.
A. (F) about 5 mm above the stylomastoid foramen
B. (T)
C. (F) the mandibular branch passes just behind the angle. 2.5 cm behind the angle is a good site for surgical incisions in order to avoid cutting this branch that supplies quadratus labii inferioris
D. (T)
E. (F) the mastoid antrum and air cells lie posterior to the nerve

61.
A. (F) the lateral aspect is affected
B. (F)
C. (F) the plantar flexors are weak and wasted
D. (T)
E. (F) the ankle jerk is impaired

62.
A. (T)
B. (F) it is not applied to the oesophagus, but separated from it by about 10 mm
C. (T) this is the aim of the operation
D. (F) tries to avoid this
E. (F) this may be performed in truncal vagotomy to aid emptying of the atonic stomach

63.
A. (T) dividing into left and right branches
B. (F) 'M' represents the coeliac axis arising from the aorta. It gives rise to the splenic artery 'O'
C. (F) 'P' is the spleen
'Q' is the left kidney
D. (T)

E. (F) it lies higher. The coeliac axis usually arises at the level of the thoraco-lumbar junction

Some of the other structures shown in this scan include: the aorta (R); the pancreas (D); the left adrenal gland (Z); and posterior vertebral muscles (X)

64.
- A. (F) at the level of L1 (first lumbar vertebra)
- B. (F) the cannula traverses: 1) skin, 2) dartos, 3) membranous layer of superficial fascia, 4) external spermatic fascia, 5) cremasteric fascia, 6) internal spermatic fascia, 7) parietal layer of tunica vaginalis (but not the visceral layer)
- C. (T)
- D. (T)
- E. (F) the left testicular vein joins the left renal vein

65.
- A. (T)
- B. (F) the azygos tributaries anastomose with the tributaries of the left gastric vein which drains into the portal vein (portal-systemic anastomosis)
- C. (F) lies anterior to the oesophagus
- D. (T)
- E. (F) about 50% of carcinomas occur in the middle third. The remainder is equally divided between the other two thirds

66.
- A. (F) it is the widest part
- B. (T)
- C. (T) therefore it is principally affected in benign prostatic hypertrophy
- D. (T)
- E. (F) only the posterior parts of the lateral lobes and the posterior lobe in the furrows between them can be palpated

67.
- A. (T) intestinal glands
- B. (F) the submucosa is highly vascular
- C. (T)
- D. (F) the inner layer is circular and the outer layer is longitudinal
- E. (F) this is a feature of an acutely inflamed appendix

68.
- A. (T)
- B. (F) the nuclei of these ductal cells are centrally located
- C. (F) this is seen in pleomorphic adenoma 'the mixed parotid tumour'
- D. (F) this is a feature of adenoid cystic carcinoma
- E. (T) it is partly serous gland

69.
- A. (T) this is important in resisting infection
- B. (F) the phrenic nerve supplying the centre of the diaphragmatic peritoneum has the same segmental origin as the supraclavicular nerve supplying the skin over the shoulder. Therefore a subphrenic abscess may cause pain over the shoulder
- C. (T)
- D. (F) the visceral peritoneum lacks sensory innervation

E. (T) this is why peritoneal dialysis for acute renal failure is possible

70.
A. (T) so does the thickness of the muscular wall
B. (T)
C. (F)
D. (F)
E. (T)

71.
A. (T)
B. (T) this anomaly is important surgically. Should the duct be ligatured jaundice will result
C. (F) it is about 6 mm on ultrasonography and about 8 mm on cholangiography
D. (T) this is of value in the recognition of the CBD
E. (F) the rectus is divided

72.
A. (F)
B. (T)
C. (T)
D. (T)
E. (F)

(See Figure 5)

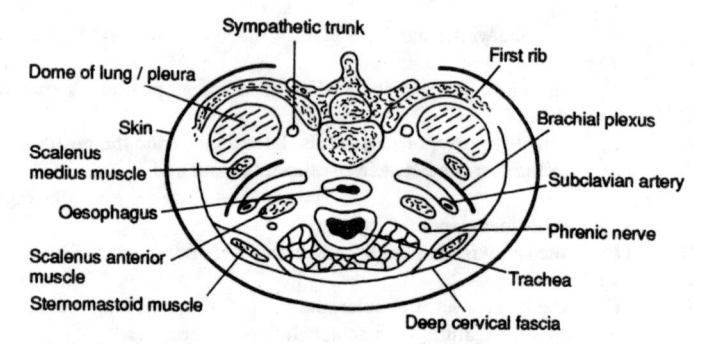

Figure 5. A transverse section through the root of the neck

73.
A. (T) a double sheet of peritoneum that folds back upon itself
B. (T) e.g. appendicitis, cholecystitis
C. (T) this may result in internal herniation of small bowel
D. (F) by gastroepiploic arteries
E. (F) anterior

74.
A. (F) the CSF is contained in the subarachnoid space
B. (F) at the level of vertebral body T9
C. (F) in the posterior white column
D. (F) the paralysis is ipsilateral
E. (T)

ANATOMY

75.
- A. (F)
- B. (F) the inferior third has no peritoneal covering
- C. (T)
- D. (F) this fascia is more developed in the male. It must be identified clearly during surgery in that region
- E. (F) the middle rectal artery is a branch of the internal iliac artery and the inferior rectal artery is a branch of the internal pudendal artery

76.
- A. (T)
- B. (F) the primary nerve supply is the accessory nerve. It also receives branches from C2 and C3
- C. (T) damage to these veins during parturition may cause a fibrosed haematoma in the lower part of the muscle (sternocleidomastoid tumour) or in severe cases torticollis due to shortening of the muscle heads
- D. (F) flex the neck anteriorly
- E. (T)

77.
- A. (T)
- B. (T) it occasionally joins the left renal vein directly
- C. (F) the cortex is mesodermal whereas the medulla arises from the neuroectoderm
- D. (T)
- E. (F) the right is usually more difficult to explore and remove because of its close relationship to the right lobe of the liver and inferior vena cava

78.
- A. (T)
- B. (F) anastomoses are seen at the lower end of the oesophagus
- C. (T) between the superior rectal veins (portal) and the middle and inferior rectal veins (systemic)
- D. (T) between the diaphragmatic veins (systemic) and liver veins (portal)
- E. (F)

79.
- A. (F)
- B. (T) damage to this vein when exposing the femoral artery may result in severe haemorrhage
- C. (F)
- D. (F) from the posterolateral aspect
- E. (F)

See Figure 6 which illustrates some of the contents of the femoral triangle

80.
- A. (T)
- B. (T) submental trauma may result in swelling in the suprahyoid region
- C. (F) the carotid sheath is formed by the visceral part of the deep cervical fascia
- D. (T) this supplies platysma

E. (F) lies deep to the deep cervical fascia

81.
A. (F) lies deep to the internal intercostal muscles
B. (F) in the subcostal groove behind the inferior border of the rib
C. (F) are branches of the internal thoracic arteries
D. (T)
E. (F)

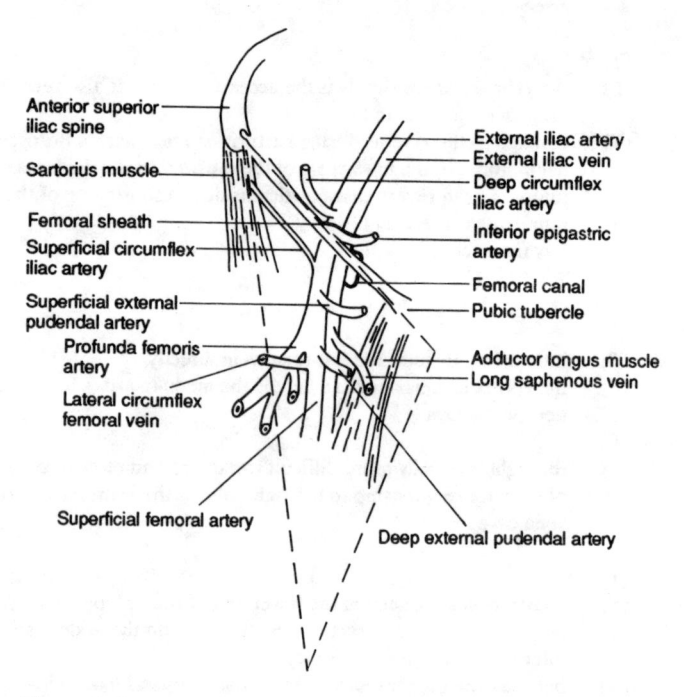

Figure 6. Contents of the right femoral triangle (- - -) underneath the fascia lata of the thigh

Labels in figure:
- Anterior superior iliac spine
- Sartorius muscle
- Femoral sheath
- Superficial circumflex iliac artery
- Superficial external pudendal artery
- Profunda femoris artery
- Lateral circumflex femoral vein
- Superficial femoral artery
- External iliac artery
- External iliac vein
- Deep circumflex iliac artery
- Inferior epigastric artery
- Femoral canal
- Pubic tubercle
- Adductor longus muscle
- Long saphenous vein
- Deep external pudendal artery

82.
A. (T)
B. (F) the pharyngeal pouch usually develops in the potential gap between the upper oblique and the lower horizontal fibres of the inferior constrictor muscle
C. (T) through the auditory tubes
D. (F) bounded by the thyroid cartilage laterally and by the aryepiglottic folds medially
E. (F) they are largest in early childhood and start to atrophy after puberty

83.
A. (T)
B. (T)
C. (F) these are supplied by the median nerve

	D.	(F)	innervated by the median nerve
	E.	(T)	
84.	A.	(F)	the lienorenal ligament transmits the splenic blood supply
	B.	(T)	this tail can be damaged at splenectomy
	C.	(T)	the spleen may be damaged when mobilizing the splenic flexure to which the ligament is attached
	D.	(T)	two segments are found in 80% of subjects three segments are found in 20% of subjects
	E.	(T)	
85.	A.	(T)	
	B.	(F)	usually deep to this muscle
	C.	(T)	this makes it essential to remove the gland during lymph nodes dissection in that region for malignancy
	D.	(T)	infection may spread from the floor of the mouth to the submandibular region (Ludwig's angina)
	E.	(T)	
86.	A.	(F)	T10
	B.	(T)	below the level of the umbilicus, lymphatics drain into the superficial inguinal group
	C.	(T)	
	D.	(F)	this space does not open into the thigh as the membranous fascia (Scarpa's fascia) is attached to fascia lata. Therefore extravasation of urine (due to rupture of penile urethra) extends up the abdominal wall deep to Scarpa's fascia and not into the thigh
	E.	(F)	a patent urachus may result in the passage of urine through the umbilicus if there is a urethral obstruction (e.g. enlarged prostate)

An umbilical faecal fistula may result from the persistence of the vitello-intestinal duct

87.	A.	(F)	'X' represents the external sphincter. 'Z' represents the internal sphincter
	B.	(T)	
	C.	(F)	just above the line
	D.	(T)	
	E.	(F)	the mucosa below the line drains into the inguinal nodes
88.	A.	(F)	Rathke's pouch gives rise to the anterior lobe
	B.	(F)	ADH is synthesized by the hypothalamus but secreted by the posterior lobe
	C.	(T)	
	D.	(T)	
	E.	(F)	the nerve passes in the lateral wall of the sinus

89.
- A. (T)
- B. (F) passes superficial to the masseter. This makes it susceptible to damage in facial injuries
- C. (T) this limits the swelling in parotitis
- D. (F) via the auriculotemporal nerve. In Frey's syndrome, where the injured auriculotemporal nerve joins the distal end of the great auricular nerve that supplies the sweat glands in the facial skin, eating stimulates sweating over the gland rather than salivation
- E. (T)

90.
- A. (T)
- B. (F)
- C. (T)
- D. (T)
- E. (T)

Figure 7 illustrates the tributaries of the long saphenous vein in the femoral triangle

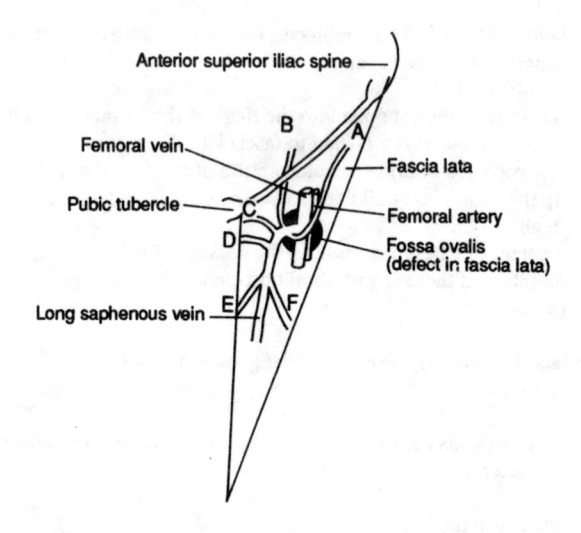

Femoral triangle showing entrance of the long saphenous vein through the fossa ovalis into the femoral vein. Tributaries of the long saphenous vein:
A = superficial circumflex iliac; B = superficial epigastric; C = superficial external pudendal; D = deep external pudendal; E = medial femoral; F = lateral femoral

Figure 7

ANATOMY

91.
- A. (F) pupil dilation results. This is because the parasympathetic fibres that supply the constrictor pupillae are interrupted
- B. (T) due to paralysis of levator palpebrae superioris
- C. (T) the superior oblique and lateral rectus are not affected
- D. (F) the afferent pathway consists of the optic nerve, optic chiasma and optic tract. The impulses pass to the oculomotor nuclei in the midbrain on both sides; the efferent pathway consists of the opposite oculomotor nerve which is intact
- E. (T) the efferent pathway is interrupted

92.
- A. (F) the absence of ionizing radiation makes MRI particularly safe
- B. (T)
- C. (T)
- D. (T)
- E. (F) CT imaging depends upon the differential absorption of radiation by the different tissue types

93.
- A. (F) it may be retracted laterally
- B. (F) the more lateral the paramedian incision the greater the risk of damaging nerve supply
- C. (F) suturing the linea alba is more important. Otherwise an incisional hernia will ensue
- D. (F) this practice weakens the scar. Separate small incisions should be used
- E. (T)

(See Figure 7a)

Various abdominal incisions

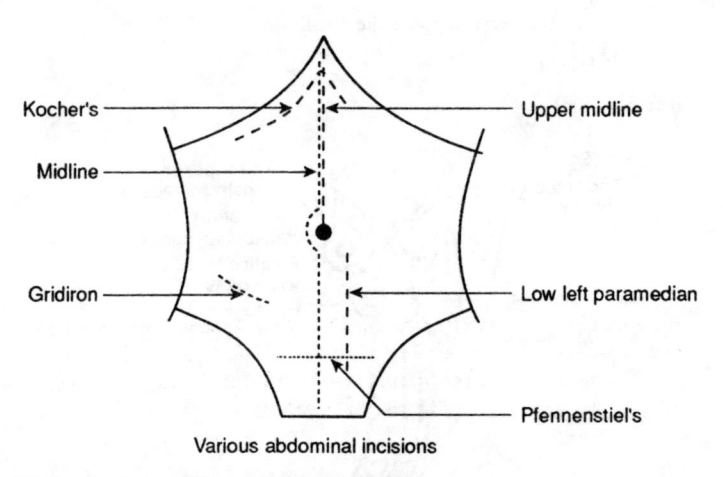

Figure 7a. Some of the abdominal incisions

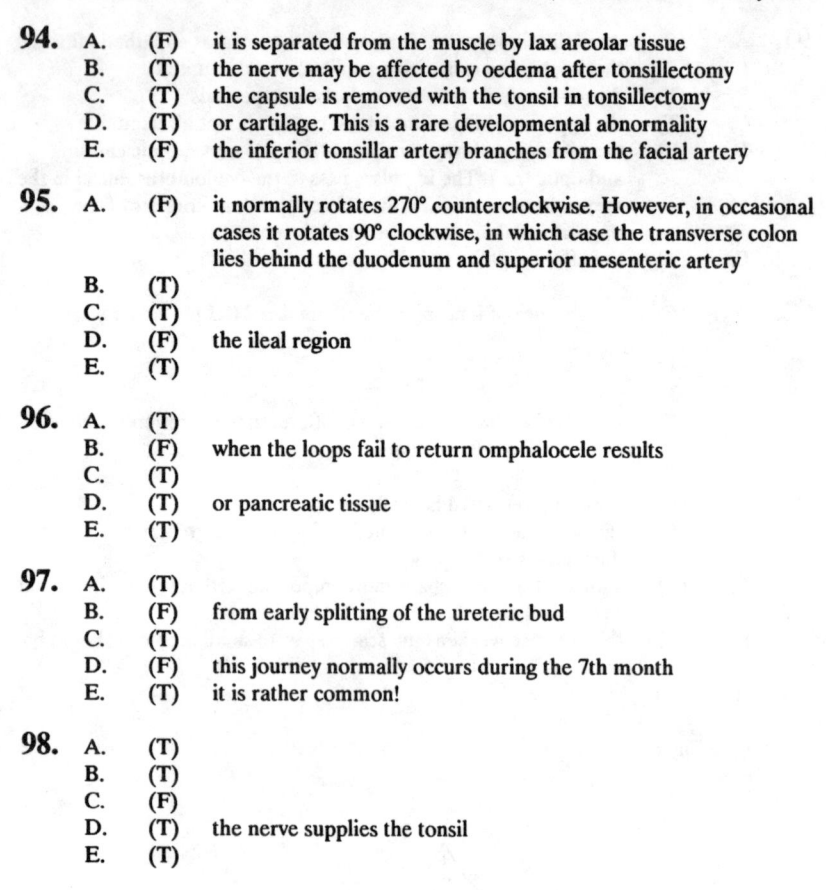

94.
- A. (F) it is separated from the muscle by lax areolar tissue
- B. (T) the nerve may be affected by oedema after tonsillectomy
- C. (T) the capsule is removed with the tonsil in tonsillectomy
- D. (T) or cartilage. This is a rare developmental abnormality
- E. (F) the inferior tonsillar artery branches from the facial artery

95.
- A. (F) it normally rotates 270° counterclockwise. However, in occasional cases it rotates 90° clockwise, in which case the transverse colon lies behind the duodenum and superior mesenteric artery
- B. (T)
- C. (T)
- D. (F) the ileal region
- E. (T)

96.
- A. (T)
- B. (F) when the loops fail to return omphalocele results
- C. (T)
- D. (T) or pancreatic tissue
- E. (T)

97.
- A. (T)
- B. (F) from early splitting of the ureteric bud
- C. (T)
- D. (F) this journey normally occurs during the 7th month
- E. (T) it is rather common!

98.
- A. (T)
- B. (T)
- C. (F)
- D. (T) the nerve supplies the tonsil
- E. (T)

(see Figure 8)

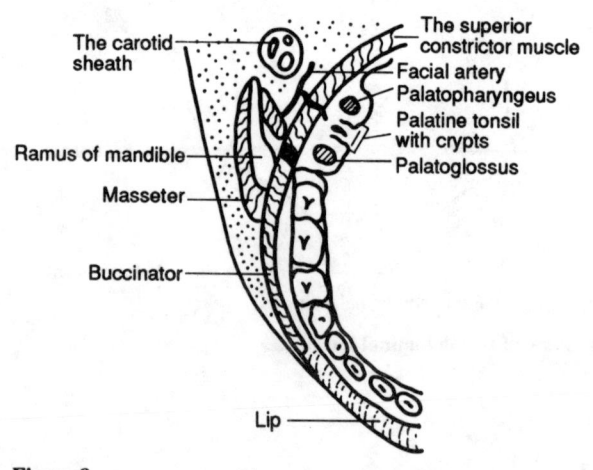

Figure 8

99.
- A. (T)
- B. (F) incomplete fusion of the trunco-conal ridges leads to a patent ductus arteriosus
- C. (T)
- D. (F) leads to right ventricular hypertrophy and underdevelopment of the left ventricle
- E. (T)

100.
- A. (F) arises from epithelial proliferation at the base of the pharynx
- B. (T) calcitonin producing cells
- C. (T)
- D. (T)
- E. (T)

Physiology and Biochemistry

1. The acute blood loss of 1.5 litres leads to a decrease in

   A. the rate of oxygen extraction by peripheral tissues
   B. the transit time of the red blood cell through the pulmonary circulation
   C. renin secretion
   D. platelet count
   E. the cardiac output

2. The acute loss of 1.5 litres of blood in a trauma patient leads to

   A. increased firing of carotid and aortic basoreceptors
   B. decreased coronary and cerebral blood flow due to sympathetic overactivity
   C. increased parasympathetic outflow to the heart
   D. only a slight decrease in mean arterial pressure (MAP)
   E. movement of intestinal fluid into capillaries

3. The consequences of biventricular failure include

   A. increased sympathetic outflow to the failing heart
   B. increased venous pressure
   C. decreased activity of renin-angiotensin-aldosterone system
   D. shifting of normal Starling curve in an upward direction
   E. accumulation of salt and water in the interstitial space

4. The effects of positive pressure ventilation (PPV) used in anaesthesia include

   A. decreased cardiac output
   B. increased pulmonary vascular resistance
   C. decreased functional residual capacity
   D. increased ADH and aldosterone secretion
   E. respiratory alkalosis

5. With respect to control of respiration

   A. the inspiratory neurons are located in the midbrain
   B. hypoxia increases the firing of the carotid bodies
   C. increased arterial PCO_2 increases ventilation mainly by stimulating the central chemoreceptors
   D. an increase in arterial H^+ concentration not due to increased PCO_2 increases ventilation mainly by stimulating the central chemoreceptors
   E. in patients with chronic obstructive airways disease hypoxia rather than hypercapnia is the main stimulus to ventilation

PHYSIOLOGY AND BIOCHEMISTRY

6. The statements below refer to the effects of a general anaesthetic (GA) on respiratory function

   A. the minute volume of ventilation is usually reduced
   B. if the cardiac output decreases, the physiological dead space increases
   C. the functional residual capacity (FRC) usually increases
   D. the lung compliance usually increases
   E. the GA does not affect the ventilation–perfusion ratio (V/Q)

7. Airflow limitation leads to a reduction in

   A. the forced expiratory volume in one second (FEV_1)
   B. the ratio of FEV_1 to forced vital capacity (FVC)
   C. lung volumes
   D. the ventilation perfusion ratio (i.e. V/Q<1)
   E. the peak expiratory flow rate (PEFR)

8. The following statements concern some investigations used in respiratory disease

   A. when performing a perfusion scan, macro-aggregated labelled human albumin remains in the pulmonary capillaries for a few hours
   B. xenon-133 gas can be used to perform a ventilation scan
   C. the gas transfer factor reflects the uptake of O_2 from the alveolus into the red cell
   D. the gas transfer factor is independent of the thickness of the alveolar membrane
   E. the gas transfer factor is usually increased in severe emphysema

9. Consider an alveolar–capillary interface. The ventilation to perfusion ratio (V/Q) is reduced if this unit is involved in

   A. pulmonary embolism
   B. pulmonary arteritis
   C. asthma
   D. lung collapse
   E. emphysema

10. With respect to respiratory function tests

   A. the peak expiratory flow rate (PEFR) in an asthmatic patient (no medication) is higher in the early morning than in the evening
   B. men have a higher PEFR than women
   C. the vitalograph spirometer measures both the forced expiratory volume in one second (FEV_1) and the forced vital capacity (FVC)
   D. recording the vitalograph involves a maximum inspiration followed by a forced expiration lasting for one second
   E. the ratio of FEV_1 to FVC is around 75% in a healthy adult

11. Consider the following diagram representing subdivisions of the lung volume (Figure 9)

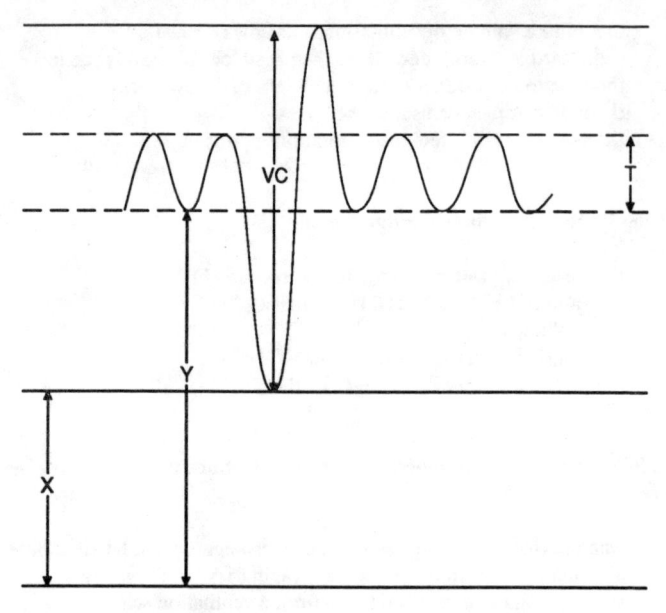

Figure 9

T = resting tidal volume; VC = vital capacity; TLC = total lung capacity; X and Y represent volumes

A. X is the functional residual capacity
B. Y is the expiratory reserve volume
C. TLC can be measured using a simple spirometer
D. a general anaesthetic increases Y
E. X is increased in a patient with emphysema

12. Considering the ABO and rhesus (Rh) systems

A. if the patient's blood group is AB, his serum will have the naturally occurring anti-A and anti-B antibodies
B. naturally occurring anti-A and anti-B antibodies are usually IgG
C. red blood cells are the only carriers of the antigens A, B and H
D. the presence of the D antigen makes the subject rhesus positive
E. rhesus antibodies are naturally occurring antibodies

13. With respect to erythropoiesis and erythropoietin

A. hypoxia is the main stimulus to erythropoietin production
B. bilateral nephrectomy completely abolishes erythropoietin activity
C. erythropoietin increases the maturation time of red blood cell precursors
D. erythropoietin stimulates ALA synthetase activity in red blood cell precursors
E. erythropoietin levels are found to be low in polycythaemia rubra vera

14. Considering the peripheral circulation and blood pressure control

A. the arterioles account for about 40% of total peripheral resistance
B. carotid chemoreceptors have no role to play in blood pressure control
C. the central vasomotor centre is situated in the medulla oblongata
D. the sudden assumption of upright posture increases discharges from the carotid and aortic baroreceptors
E. the sudden assumption of upright posture causes constriction of medium sized veins

15. The extrinsic pathway of the coagulation cascade involves the following factors

A. tissue factor
B. factor VII
C. factor IX
D. Ca^{2+}
E. factor XI

16. Considering vitamin K

A. fat malabsorption is the commonest cause of vitamin K deficiency in adults
B. none of the available preparations can be absorbed in the absence of bile salts
C. vitamin dependent factors require the vitamin for carboxylation of their N-terminal residues so that they can chelate calcium
D. vitamin K reverses warfarin effects almost instantaneously
E. warfarin inhibits the reduction of 2,3 epoxide to quinone

17. Following trauma to a blood vessel

A. the platelets immediately adhere to subendothelial fibres
B. platelet aggregation is induced by ADP and thrombin
C. serotonin (5HT) is released by the granules of the platelet release reactions
D. the vessel wall endothelium produces thromboxane A_2 which inhibits platelet adhesion
E. low dose aspirin does not affect the synthesis of thromboxane A_2

18. The following occur in the successfully sympathectomized left hand

A. permanent abolition of sweating
B. the skin does not respond to central temperature changes
C. the skin does not respond to local temperature changes
D. the large increase in blood flow following the operation is well maintained for years
E. if the skin is ischaemic, the ischaemia may improve

19. The following factors stimulate ADH (vasopressin) secretion

A. exercise
B. alcohol
C. severe hypovolaemia
D. decreased plasma osmolarity
E. pain

20. The following statements concern bilirubin and its metabolites

A. the daily production of bilirubin in a 70 kg adult is about 300 mg
B. the conjugation of bilirubin is performed by the enzymes β-glucuronidases
C. the conjugated bilirubin is secreted into the bile by simple diffusion
D. a fraction of urobilinogen is re-absorbed from the intestine and re-excreted through the liver
E. urobilins are colourless compounds

21. With respect to potassium haemostasis in the body

A. 30% of the total body potassium is located in the extracellular compartment
B. aldosterone increases active potassium secretion in the distal convoluted tubule
C. hypokalaemia directly stimulates aldosterone secretion
D. hypokalaemia will ensue if the activity of the membrane-bound, ATP-dependent sodium pump is impaired
E. insulin causes potassium to enter the cell]

22. The following statements concern CO_2 in the blood

A. for a given pH, the partial pressure of CO_2 (PCO_2) is inversely proportional to bicarbonate concentration [HCO_3]
B. most of the CO_2 in the blood is present in the form of carbonic acid H_2CO_3
C. CO_2 diffuses into red blood cells in the capillary beds
D. haemoglobin is the main buffer for H^+ generated by the entry of CO_2 into red blood cells
E. PCO_2 is usually higher than normal in compensated metabolic alkalosis

PHYSIOLOGY AND BIOCHEMISTRY

23. With respect to hydrogen ion homeostasis (H^+)

- A. bicarbonate is the most important buffer in the extracellular fluid
- B. proteins are the principal buffer in urine
- C. hydrogen ions are secreted into the renal tubular lumen in exchange for potassium ions (K^+), so that they combine with the filtered bicarbonate
- D. ammonium ions (NH_4^+) can cross the membranes of renal tubular cells
- E. the hydrogen ion concentration is directly proportional to the partial pressure of CO_2

24. When measuring the GFR in a potential kidney donor

- A. creatinine clearance is higher than the true GFR
- B. creatinine clearance is directly proportional to serum creatinine concentration
- C. the GFR can be calculated from the rate of fall of serum radioactivity after the injection of ^{51}Cr-labelled EDTA
- D. serum urea is a more accurate index of GFR than serum creatinine
- E. insulin clearance is used to estimate GFR in routine clinical practice

25. With respect to the nephron in a healthy kidney

- A. the descending loop of Henle is impermeable to water
- B. almost all the filtered protein is re-absorbed in the proximal convoluted tubule
- C. ADH renders the cells lining the collecting ducts permeable to water
- D. in the distal tubule, further Na^+ is re-absorbed while K^+ and H^+ are secreted under the influence of ADH (vasopressin)
- E. all the filtered glucose is re-absorbed in the proximal tubule

26. The following provide a reasonably good assessment of GFR

- A. serum albumin
- B. serum creatinine
- C. serum β_2-microglobulin (in a healthy subject)
- D. water deprivation test
- E. amino acid chromatography on urine

27. The following are increased by hypoglycaemia

- A. glucagon secretion
- B. epinephrine output from the adrenal medulla
- C. glucokinase activity
- D. growth hormone secretion by the anterior pituitary
- E. cortisol secretion

28. Regarding the citric acid cycle

A. acetyl-CoA combines with oxaloacetate to form citrate
B. hypoxia stimulates the cycle
C. vitamin B_1 (thiamin) plays a role in the functioning of the cycle
D. eleven ATP molecules are produced per turn of the cycle
E. the cycle acts as the final common pathway for lipids, proteins and carbohydrates

29. The following factors inhibit gastric acid secretion

A. histamine
B. H_1-blockers
C. gastrin inhibiting polypeptide (GIP)
D. atropine
E. gastrin

30. Twenty-four hours after a haemorrhagic shock the plasma level of the following hormones is found to be increased

A. cortisol
B. insulin
C. adrenalin
D. growth hormone
E. noradrenaline

31. The following metabolic changes occur in the EBB phase (first 24 hours) of response to injury

A. plasma pH increases
B. the plasma level of free fatty acid decreases
C. hypoglycaemia
D. the plasma level of non-protein nitrogen decreases
E. plasma glycerol increases

32. On the fourth day following major surgery the plasma level of the following proteins is found to be increased

A. α_1 globulin
B. albumin
C. transferrin
D. α_2 globulin
E. β-lipoprotein

33. Considering complete acute obstruction of the small intestine

A. initially there is intermittent colicky pain which is sharply localized
B. the gas in the distended bowel is mainly due to methane and hydrogen disulphide produced in the intestine
C. the flux of fluids and electrolytes from the lumen back into the tissues is markedly reduced in the obstructed segment
D. the obstructed segment provides a good environment for bacterial proliferation
E. the intraluminal pressure does not exceed 10 cm of water

34. Considering the physiology of the small intestine

A. about 9 litres of secretions enter the upper part of the intestine in a healthy subject every day
B. the absorption of water is mainly a passive process
C. the vitamin B_{12}-intrinsic factor complex enters the mucosal cells of the terminal ileum after binding to specific receptors
D. the principal action of pancreatic lipase is to convert triglycerides to glycerol and fatty acids
E. bile salts are absorbed into the mucosal cells along with the products of fat digestion

35. Motility of the small intestine may be reduced by

A. neostigmine
B. abdominal exploration
C. morphine
D. vagotomy
E. excessive hydroxytryptamine secretion in the carcinoid syndrome

36. Vasopressin (ADH)

A. is synthesized in the posterior pituitary gland
B. deficiency leads to a risk of water intoxication
C. excessive secretion usually results in diabetes insipidus (DI)
D. increased plasma osmolarity is the primary physiological stimulus
E. acts mainly on the distal convoluted tubules and collecting ducts of the kidney

37. Human growth hormone (hGH)

A. is synthesized by basophilic cells in the anterior pituitary
B. secretion is stimulated by a rise in blood glucose concentration
C. the growth related effects are primarily mediated by somatomedin C
D. secretion is inhibited by somatostatin
E. increases protein synthesis

38. **The following diagram represents the haemoglobin–oxygen dissociation curve (Figure 10)**

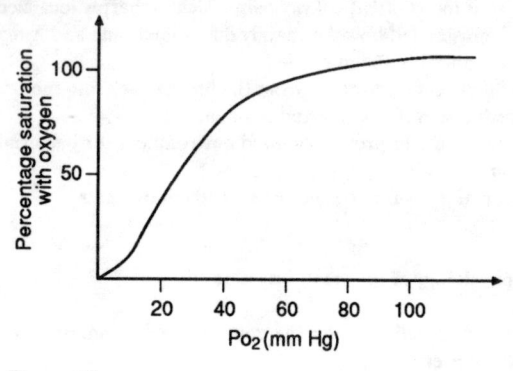

Figure 10

The curve is shifted to the right in:

A. pyrexia
B. respiratory acidosis
C. states of decreased concentration of 2,3 DPG inside the red cell
D. polycythaemia
E. sickle cell anaemia

39. **Considering hormones and pregnancy**

A. human chorionic gonadotrophin (hCG) becomes undetectable in urine in the third trimester
B. the synthesis of human placental lactogen (hPL) is dependent upon both placental and foetal enzymes
C. pregnanediol is the main urinary metabolite of progesterone
D. a low serum progesterone in pregnancy is associated with recurrent abortions
E. the foetal liver and adrenals take part in the synthesis of oestriol

40. **The principal actions of insulin include**

A. increased lipolysis in adipose tissue
B. increased ketogenesis in the liver
C. increased glucose uptake by muscle and adipose tissue
D. decreased glycogen synthesis
E. increased protein synthesis

41. With respect to bile

A. about 2 litres of bile are secreted into the duodenum daily
B. most of the bile acids are reabsorbed in the colon
C. some of the urobilinogen absorbed in the colon is excreted in the urine
D. the solubility of cholesterol in the bile is independent of its relative molar concentration
E. cholecystokinin–pancreozymin causes bile secretion into the duodenum

42. The following statements concern the cardioplegic solution and myocardial protection when the aorta is cross clamped proximal to the coronary arteries in a cardiac operation

A. the myocardium can survive this ischaemia for about 25 minutes, even if the cardioplegic solution has not been used
B. the cardioplegic solution may contain histidine buffers which bind to harmful compounds
C. when injected into the coronary arteries the cardioplegic solution has a temperature of 20°C
D. the cardioplegic solution contains potassium and procaine which cause a rapid cardiac arrest
E. when the cardioplegic solution is used, the heart can easily survive ischaemia for about 10 hours

43. The following statements concern thyroid hormones (T_3 and T_4) in a healthy subject

A. they are principally bound to albumin
B. the concentration of free T_4 is greater than that of T_3
C. T_3 has a half life of 7 days
D. an increase in the concentration of the binding protein leads to stimulation of TSH secretion
E. they bind to nuclear receptors to stimulate the synthesis of mRNA

44. With respect to calcium homeostasis

A. about 99% of the body calcium is bound to the skeleton
B. the ionized calcium concentration in the plasma increases in acute alkalosis
C. clinical chemistry laboratories usually measure and report the ionized calcium concentration
D. calcitonin stimulates bone resorption
E. PTH stimulates 1α-hydroxylation of 25-hydroxycholecalciferol in the kidneys

45. Pancreatic secretion (exocrine) may be stimulated by

  A. gastrin
  B. secretin
  C. atropine
  D. cholecystokinin–pancreozymin (CCK–PZ)
  E. vasoactive intestinal polypeptide (VIP)

46. The following statements concern the basic heart–lung bypass circuit

  A. the oxygenator should be about 20" above the level of the patient
  B. the circuit has a capacity of 2.5 litres
  C. there is an initial haemodilation when the bypass circuit is connected to the patient
  D. the intra-aortic pressure is usually insufficient to keep the aortic valve closed
  E. the patient is usually heparinized

47. Considering ammonia

  A. glutamine formation is the major pathway of ammonia removal by the liver
  B. renal veins have higher ammonia levels than the renal arteries
  C. ammonia production by the kidneys is decreased in metabolic acidosis
  D. the brain cannot convert ammonia to urea
  E. the portal venous blood has a higher ammonia concentration than that of the systemic blood

48. The effects of glucocorticoids include

  A. increasing prostaglandin synthesis
  B. decreasing the number of circulating leucocytes
  C. increasing the delivery of amino acids to the liver to increase glucose production
  D. suppression of the immune response
  E. potassium reabsorption in the distal renal tubule

49. When the renin–angiotensin–aldosterone system is stimulated by a hypovolaemic shock

  A. renin converts angiotensin I to angiotensin II
  B. angiotensin II causes vasoconstriction of the efferent glomerular arteriole
  C. angiotensin II stimulates the adrenal medulla to synthesize aldosterone
  D. angiotensin II stimulates the adrenal cortex to increase cortisol production
  E. angiotensin converting enzymes degrade bradykinin

50. The following factors stimulate renin release

- A. a decrease in blood pressure
- B. propranolol
- C. an increase in plasma K^+ concentration
- D. angiotensin II
- E. salt depletion

51. The blood-brain barrier (BBB)

- A. contains endothelial cells which have tight junctions
- B. allows transport of substances in one direction only, i.e. out of the vascular system into the brain
- C. allows water to cross by simple diffusion
- D. contains astrocytic foot processes
- E. lacks mitochondria in the endothelial cells

52. The normal CSF contains

- A. about 10 polymorphs per mm^3
- B. oligoclonal bands in 50% of cases
- C. 0.2–0.4 mg of protein per litre
- D. immunoglobulins (IgG)
- E. less than 1/3 of blood glucose

53. The diagram below represents an action potential recorded from an unmyelinated axon (Figure 11)

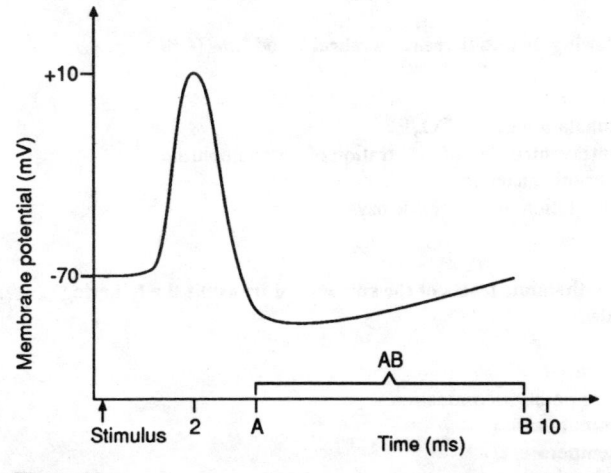

Figure 11

A. during the period AB (hyperpolarization) the Na$^+$-channels are more active than the K$^+$ channels
B. during AB a stronger current (stimulus) is needed to generate another action potential
C. more ionic exchange (across the membrane) occurs in this unmyelinated axon than in a myelinated axon
D. the greater the diameter of the axon the greater the conduction velocity of this action potential
E. saltatory conduction is a feature of conduction in unmyelinated axons

54. The electromyogram (EMG)

A. records the electrical activity of muscle fibres making up the motor units
B. records the magnitude of muscle contraction
C. shows regular electrical activity when healthy muscle is relaxed
D. can be recorded by placing the electrode on the skin overlying the muscle
E. shows fibrillation potentials in denervated muscle

55. The following statements are true

A. midcollicular section causes decerebrate rigidity
B. midcollicular section causes the EEG to become fast, low in amplitude and desynchronized
C. midpontine section causes decerebrate rigidity
D. high spinal section leaves the isolated brain with a normal sleep/waking EEG cycle
E. midpontine section causes the EEG to show slow high-amplitude activity that is synchronized as in sleep

56. The following factors decrease cerebral blood flow (CBF)

A. seizures
B. inhalation of 7% CO_2
C. intraventricular administration of norepinephrine
D. chronic anaemia
E. inhalation of hyperbaric oxygen

57. The spinothalamic tracts of the spinal cord transmit the following sensory modalities

A. pain
B. two point discrimination
C. joint position
D. temperature
E. vibration

58. The following autonomic neurons are adrenergic

   A. postganglion sympathetic neuron to the small bowel
   B. postganglion sympathetic neurons to the sweat gland
   C. some preganglionic neurons
   D. the parasympathetic fibres supplying the sphincter pupillae of the iris
   E. postganglionic parasympathetic neurons to the stomach

59. Cholinergic impulses in the autonomic nervous system produce

   A. a decrease in atrial contractility
   B. detrusor muscle relaxation
   C. ciliary muscle contraction
   D. gallbladder relaxation
   E. ejaculation

60. The following factors stimulate gastrin secretion

   A. increased vagal activity
   B. hypercalcaemia
   C. increased gastric acidity
   D. secretin
   E. a protein meal

61. The diagram below shows the various parts of the electrocardiogram (Figure 12)

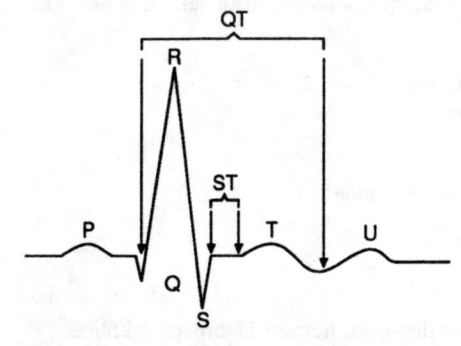

Figure 12

The following statements are correct

   A. opening of the aortic valve coincides with the P wave
   B. isovolumetric contraction occurs during the P wave
   C. during the ST segments all parts of ventricles have been depolarized
   D. the QT interval may be prolonged in hypokalaemia
   E. during the T wave, the tricuspid valve is normally closed

62. The following are non-operative methods for reducing intracranial pressure

A. hypoventilation
B. intravenous mannitol
C. the administration of atracurium
D. the administration of sodium nitroprusside
E. positioning the patient in the head down position

63. The following transmitter substances increase intestinal secretion of water and electrolytes

A. noradrenaline
B. VIP (vasoactive intestinal polypeptide)
C. prostaglandins
D. dihydroxy bile acids
E. acetylcholine

64. In the digestion and absorption of fat

A. the mixed micelle formed is water-soluble
B. vitamins K, D, A and E are packaged into the chylomicrons within the enterocytes
C. most of the chylomicrons pass from the enterocytes into the portal vein
D. deficiency of apoprotein B synthesis causes fat malabsorption
E. long-chain triglycerides are more water-soluble than medium-chain triglycerides (MCTs)

65. Within the first week post-injury in a severely traumatized patient, there is increased

A. secretion of aldosterone
B. excretion of urea in urine
C. protein synthesis
D. lipolysis
E. anti-diuretic hormone secretion

66. Nociception (pain)

A. is transmitted faster through C fibres than through AΔ fibres
B. does not ascend through the dorsal column of the spinal cord
C. in disseminated cancer, may be effectively relieved by intracranial morphine
D. transmission is facilitated by the stimulation of μ receptors in the CNS
E. in disseminated cancer, may be relieved by hypophysectomy

PHYSIOLOGY AND BIOCHEMISTRY

67. The cerebral blood flow (CBF)

- A. accounts for about 15% of the cardiac output
- B. is decreased by hypocapnia
- C. is decreased by hypoxia
- D. is mainly controlled by sympathetic and parasympathetic mechanism
- E. is increased by isoflorane in general anaesthesia

68. The following factors usually depress the cardiac output (CO)

- A. intravenous thiopentone
- B. a high dose of methohexitone
- C. hypothermia
- D. moderate anaemia
- E. atropine administration

69. The colonic epithelium

- A. is an important site for potassium absorption
- B. absorbs chloride in exchange for bicarbonate
- C. absorbs sodium in linkage with glucose via an active carrier-mediated mechanism
- D. rate of sodium absorption is influenced by aldosterone
- E. absorbs carbohydrates mainly in the form of short-chain fatty acids

70. With respect to fluids used in intravenous fluid replacement

- A. dextran 40 may interfere with blood cross-matching
- B. haemaccel may cause coagulation defects
- C. plasma protein fraction (PPF) has a half-life of 12 hours
- D. plasma protein fraction commonly causes anaphylactic reactions
- E. 1 litre of normal saline (0.9% NaCl) contains about 150 millimoles of sodium

71. The actions of antidiuretic hormone (ADH) include

- A. reduction of cardiac output
- B. an increase of total peripheral resistance
- C. decreased release of ACTH
- D. increased renal reabsorption of sodium
- E. decreased release of factor VIII

72. The luteinizing hormone releasing hormone (LHRH)

A. has a constant secretion rate throughout the day
B. controls the secretion of FSH
C. analogues may be used in the treatment of prostatic carcinoma
D. may be used in the treatment of infertility in both sexes
E. produces a greater response in LH release when given (intravenously) during the early follicular phase rather than during the luteal phase

73. With respect to vomiting

A. the main receptors in the chemoreceptor trigger zone (CTZ) are dopaminergic (D2)
B. the CTZ is not protected by the blood–brain barrier
C. $5HT_3$ (hydroxytryptamine) agonists may be effective as anti-emetics in cis-platinum-induced vomiting
D. afferents from the stomach wall travel via the vagus nerve to the CTZ and vomiting centre
E. H_2 receptors are abundant in the vomiting centre

74. The following statements are correct

A. aldosterone acts on the colonic epithelium to enhance sodium absorption in exchange for K^+ and H^+
B. hyperaldosteronism is a feature of congestive heart failure
C. hyperkalaemia usually causes narrow QRS complexes and inverted T-waves in the ECG
D. hypovolaemic shock may lead to swelling of cells
E. hypercalcaemia potentiates the action of lignocaine

75. With reference to body temperature and general anaesthesia (GA)

A. the patient tends to become poikilothermic during GA
B. GA depresses the hypothalamic heat control mechanisms
C. GA increases heat production
D. malignant hyperpyrexia syndrome (MHS) has been known to be triggered by enflurane
E. MHS is characterized by hypokalaemic alkalosis

76. Total parenteral nutrition (TPN)

A. contains protein in the form of hydrolysates of casein
B. contains albumin
C. should be enriched with aromatic amino acids in patients with hepatic failure
D. may be complicated by hyperosmolar crisis
E. contains zinc and copper

Answers

1.
- A. (F) this is increased
- B. (F) this is increased
- C. (F) renin secretion is increased in response to low renal perfusion due to hypovolaemia
- D. (F) increases
- E. (T) the stroke volume falls

2.
- A. (F) the firing of these receptors decreases in response to the fall in blood pressure
- B. (F) the blood flow of these organs remains almost unchanged
- C. (F) the parasympathetic outflow to the heart decreases
- D. (T) MAP = total peripheral resistance × cardiac output
- E. (T) due to arteriolar constriction and hypotension

3.
- A. (T) to increase heart rate and myocardial contractility
- B. (T)
- C. (F) the activity increases due to decrease in renal perfusion
- D. (F) Starling curve shifts in a downward direction when the heart fails
- E. (T) producing oedema

4.
- A. (T) due to decreased venous return, depressed ventricular performance and increased pulmonary vascular resistance
- B. (T)
- C. (F) this increases by about 17%
- D. (T) due to decreased renal perfusion
- E. (T) if the patient is over-ventilated

5.
- A. (F) these neurons are located in the medulla
- B. (T) peripheral chemoreceptors
- C. (T)
- D. (F) H^+ ions penetrate the blood–barrier very poorly. They stimulate peripheral chemoreceptors
- E. (T)

6.
- A. (T) due to either a decrease in respiratory rate or a decrease in the volume of each breath
- B. (T) the gas exchange is impaired due to reduced perfusion of alveoli
- C. (F) when the subject lies down the diaphragm rises and therefore the FRC decreases
- D. (F) the compliance decreases partly due to a reduction in FRC
- E. (F) V/Q ratio is altered by the reduced cardiac output, the respiratory depression and the lying down position

7.
- A. (T)
- B. (T)
- C. (F) lung volumes are normal or increased
- D. (T)
- E. (T)

8.
- A. (T)
- B. (T)
- C. (T)
- D. (F)
- E. (F) it is usually reduced

9.
- A. (F) ventilation but no perfusion (V/Q > 1)
- B. (F) perfusion is reduced (V/Q > 1)
- C. (T)
- D. (T)
- E. (T)

10.
- A. (F) lower in the early morning (diurnal variation)
- B. (T)
- C. (T)
- D. (F) the act of expiration should continue until all the air has been expelled from the lung
- E. (T)

11.
- A. (F) X is the residual volume
- B. (F) Y is the functional residual capacity
- C. (F) by other techniques e.g. helium dilution
- D. (F) as the subject lies down the diaphragm rises, thus reducing the FRC (Y)
- E. (T)

12.
- A. (F) his serum will not have anti-A and anti-B antibodies
- B. (F) are usually IgM
- C. (F) these antigens are present on most body cells, e.g. white cells, platelets, etc.
- D. (T)
- E. (F) Rh antibodies are immune antibodies

13.
- A. (T)
- B. (F) this indicates another source for erythropoietin production, e.g. liver
- C. (F) it decreases the maturation time of these cells
- D. (T) to increase Hb synthesis
- E. (T) the elevated Hb level reduces erythropoietin synthesis

14.
- A. (T)
- B. (F) hypoxia stimulates chemoreceptors causing vasoconstriction and tachycardia through central mechanisms
- C. (T)
- D. (F) the basoreceptors discharge decreases, as these receptors are stretch receptors which are stimulated by distension of the vessels containing them
- E. (T) due to sympathetic stimulation

15.
- A. (T)
- B. (T)
- C. (F)
- D. (T)
- E. (F)

16.
- A. (T) In the neonate, vitamin K deficiency is usually due to absence of bacteria in the foetal gut able to synthesize vitamin K
- B. (F) menandione is a water-soluble form which can be absorbed in the absence of bile salts
- C. (F) factors II, VII, IX and X undergo decarboxylation in the presence of vitamin K
- D. (F) it takes about 12–20 hours to reverse warfarin anticoagulation
- E. (T)

17.
- A. (T)
- B. (T)
- C. (T)
- D. (F) these cells produce prostacyclin which inhibits platelet adhesion
- E. (F) low-dose aspirin irreversibly inhibits the process

18.
- A. (T)
- B. (T)
- C. (F)
- D. (F) the large increase is initial and within 2 weeks the blood flow falls considerably
- E. (T)

19.
- A. (T)
- B. (F) alcohol inhibits ADH secretion
- C. (T)
- D. (F) this inhibits ADH secretion
- E. (T)

20.
- A. (T) this is equivalent to 6 g of haemoglobin
- B. (F) these bacterial enzymes deconjugate bilirubin in the intestine
- C. (F) it is secreted against a concentration gradient, therefore an active transport system is required
- D. (T) (the entero-hepatic circulation)
- E. (F) urobilinogens are colourless, whereas urobilins are coloured

21.
- A. (F) only about 2% is found in this compartment
- B. (T) aldosterone also increases potassium excretion at this site by stimulating active sodium re-absorption
- C. (F) hyperkalaemia is a stimulus. Aldosterone increases potassium excretion
- D. (F) potassium will accumulate in the extracellular compartment and hyperkalaemia will ensue
- E. (T)

22.
- A. (F) $PCO_2 = pH \times K \times [HCO_3^-]$
- B. (F) in the form of bicarbonate HCO_3^-
- C. (T)
- D. (T)
- E. (T)

23.
- A. (T)
- B. (F) phosphate is the principal buffer in urine (HPO_4^{2-}). Ammonia is also important
- C. (F) they are secreted in exchange for Na^+
- D. (F) ammonia (NH_3) can
- E. (T) $[H^+] = K \dfrac{PCO_2}{[HCO_3^-]}$

24.
- A. (T) this is because creatinine is actively secreted in the renal tubules
- B. (F) (inversely proportional)
- C. (T)
- D. (F) there are many factors that influence urea production and concentration
- E. (F) creatinine clearance is preferred as inulin has to be injected into the subject. However, serum creatinine is the simplest and most widely used estimate of GFR

25.
- A. (F) the ascending loop is impermeable
- B. (T) very little protein is excreted in urine (<150 mg/day)
- C. (T) this produces a concentrated urine
- D. (F) this is controlled by aldosterone and not ADH
- E. (T)

26.
- A. (F)
- B. (T)
- C. (T)
- D. (F) this assesses distal tubular function
- E. (F) this is a test of proximal tubular function

27.
- A. (T)
- B. (T)
- C. (F) this enzyme facilitates glucose uptake by the liver, hence activity increases with hyperglycaemia
- D. (T)
- E. (T)

28.
- A. (T)
- B. (F) it partially inhibits the cycle as oxygen is required for oxidation
- C. (T) as a coenzyme
- D. (F) twelve ATP molecules are produced
- E. (T)

29.
- A. (F) this stimulates gastric acid secretion
- B. (F) these do not effect gastric acid secretion

	C.	(T)	
	D.	(T)	
	E.	(F)	this hormone stimulates gastric acid secretion
30.	A.	(T)	
	B.	(F)	this initially decreases to rise later
	C.	(T)	
	D.	(T)	
	E.	(T)	
31.	A.	(F)	there is usually acidosis, i.e. pH decreases
	B.	(F)	this usually increases due to increased lipolysis
	C.	(F)	hyperglycaemia
	D.	(F)	increases
	E.	(T)	see B
32.	A.	(T)	maximum on the third day
	B.	(F)	this usually decreases by about 25% minimum around the fourth day
	C.	(F)	this usually decreases
	D.	(T)	maximum on the third day
	E.	(F)	this usually decreases
33.	A.	(F)	the pain is not sharply localized but lies across the abdomen at the level of the umbilicus. This is because the small bowel is derived from the foregut
	B.	(F)	the gas is mainly derived from the swallowed air
	C.	(T)	Shields demonstrated this in 1965
	D.	(T)	
	E.	(F)	may rise as high as 25 cm of water
34.	A.	(T)	
	B.	(T)	due to the active absorption of the products of carbohydrate and protein digestion
	C.	(F)	the complex is split off at the brush border and only vitamin B_{12} is absorbed
	D.	(F)	lipase principally converts triglycerides into monoglycerides and fatty acids
	E.	(F)	bile salts are re-used. Re-absorption of bile salts occurs in the terminal ileum
35.	A.	(F)	this increases intestinal motility by inhibiting cholinesterase
	B.	(T)	post-operative ileus
	C.	(T)	
	D.	(T)	
	E.	(F)	diarrhoea
36.	A.	(F)	it is synthesized in the supraoptic nucleus of the hypothalamus and transported to the posterior pituitary via axoplasmic flow
	B.	(F)	excessive secretion leads to such a risk as there is impaired water

			excretion
	C.	(F)	DI results from deficient secretion or action of the hormone leading to thirst and polyuria
	D.	(T)	
	E.	(T)	

37.
	A.	(F)	by somatotropes which are a subclass of the pituitary acidophilic cells
	B.	(F)	fall in glucose concentration is a stimulus to its secretion
	C.	(T)	somatomedins are produced by the liver
	D.	(T)	
	E.	(T)	anabolic effect

38.
	A.	(T)	
	B.	(T)	
	C.	(F)	this shifts the curve to the left
	D.	(F)	
	E.	(T)	

Note: shift to right is advantageous as the blood gives up its oxygen more readily

39.
	A.	(F)	although it begins to fall around the 11th week, it remains detectable
	B.	(F)	the foetal enzymes are not involved (cf oestriol)
	C.	(T)	
	D.	(T)	
	E.	(T)	this can be used to monitor foeto-placental function

40.
	A.	(F)	decreased
	B.	(F)	decreased
	C.	(T)	
	D.	(F)	increased
	E.	(T)	anabolic effect

41.
	A.	(F)	about 500 ml
	B.	(F)	in the terminal ileum
	C.	(T)	
	D.	(F)	the solubility decreases as the relative molar concentration increases
	E.	(T)	CCK-PZ contracts the gallbladder and relaxes the sphincter of Oddi

42.
	A.	(T)	
	B.	(T)	these compounds are byproducts of ischaemia
	C.	(F)	4°C. Hypothermia decreases the metabolic rate of the myocardial cells
	D.	(T)	
	E.	(F)	10 hours is too long. The solution provides a good protection for up to 2 hours

PHYSIOLOGY AND BIOCHEMISTRY

43.
- A. (F) thyroxine binding globulin (TBG) is the principal binding protein
- B. (T)
- C. (F) T_3 has a $T_{1/2}$ of 1.5 days compared with 6–7 days for T_4
- D. (T) as (TBG) increases more T_4 binds to it, therefore the concentration of free T_4 decreases and this stimulates TSH synthesis
- E. (T) to synthesize various polypeptides

44.
- A. (T) in the form of hydroxyapatite
- B. (F) it decreases
- C. (F) usually measure the total calcium concentration. However, it is possible to measure the concentration of the ionized form using ion selective electrodes
- D. (F) calcitonin experimentally inhibits osteoclastic activity
- E. (T)

45.
- A. (T) the sequence of the 5 amino acids at the C-terminal end is identical to that of CCK-PZ
- B. (T) stimulates electrolyte secretion
- C. (F) antimuscarinic agents reduce secretion
- D. (T) it also causes gall bladder contraction
- E. (T) this is similar in structure to secretin

46.
- A. (F) the oxygenator should be lower than the patient to allow the venous blood to drain by gravity syphonage
- B. (T)
- C. (T) this is due to the added fluid present in the circuit
- D. (F)
- E. (T)

47.
- A. (F) conversion to urea is the major pathway
- B. (T) this is due to intracellular production of ammonia by renal tubules
- C. (F) it is increased (ammonia is a buffer)
- D. (F) it can, although glutamine formation is the major pathway of ammonia removal
- E. (T) due to ammonia absorbed from the gut (produced by enteric bacteria)

48.
- A. (F) glucocorticoids induce lipocortins which inhibit phospholipase A2, thus decreasing the production of prostaglandins and leucotrienes
- B. (T)
- C. (T)
- D. (T)
- E. (F) glucocorticoids cause Na^+ retention and K^+ excretion

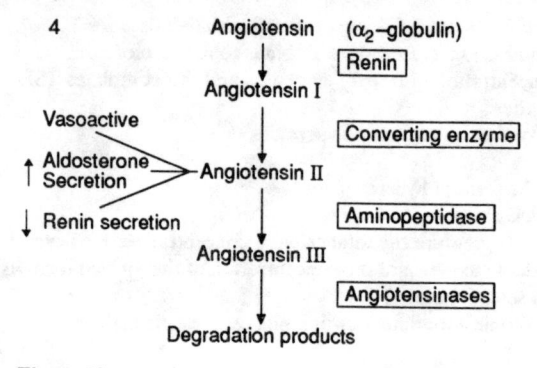

49. A. (F) angiotensin (α_2-globulin) (See Figure 13)

```
        4              Angiotensin    (α₂-globulin)
                            ↓         [Renin]
                       Angiotensin I
   Vasoactive               ↓         [Converting enzyme]
  ↑ Aldosterone
    Secretion  ╲ ╱  Angiotensin II
               ╳
  ↓ Renin secretion ╱         ↓         [Aminopeptidase]
                       Angiotensin III
                            ↓         [Angiotensinases]
                       Degradation products
```

Figure 13

B. (T)
C. (F) the adrenal cortex, not the medulla, secretes aldosterone
D. (F) angiotensin II does not affect cortisol production
E. (T) bradykinin is a vasodilator

50. A. (T)
B. (F) β-blockers inhibit renin release
C. (F) this inhibits renin release
D. (F) it inhibits renin release, forming a negative feedback mechanism
E. (T)

51. A. (T)
B. (F) the transport system may work in the opposite direction
C. (T)
D. (T)
E. (F) the BBB endothelial cells have six times the mitochondria found in endothelial cells elsewhere

52. A. (F) mononuclear cells only. No polymorphs (cell count 5/mm^3)
B. (F) these bands are usually absent. Their presence is pathologically significant, e.g. multiple sclerosis
C. (F) 0.2 – 0.4 g/L
D. (T) these constitute less than 15% of total protein
E. (F) > ½ blood glucose. A low glucose content is a feature of bacterial meningitis

53. A. (F) the K$^+$-channels are more active
B. (T)
C. (T) ionic exchange in myelinated axons occurs mainly at the nodes of Ranvier. This means that less metabolic energy is required in myelinated fibres to pump the ions out once the impulse has passed
D. (T) myelination also increases conduction velocity

PHYSIOLOGY AND BIOCHEMISTRY 69

E. (F) saltatory (Latin: saltare, to leap) conduction is a feature of myelinated fibres, where the active region leaps from one node of Ranvier to another

54. A. (T)
B. (F)
C. (F) no changes in potential are visible
D. (T) the electrode can be also inserted into muscle
E. (T)

55. A. (T) γ-efferents are facilitated
B. (F) the EEG becomes slow, large and synchronized (sleep-like)
C. (F) such a section abolishes decerebrate rigidity by removing mid-brain facilitation
D. (T)
E. (F) the cortex 'wakens' as the medullary inhibitory centres are cut off

56. A. (F) CBF increases
B. (F) CBF increases by more than 100%
C. (F) CBF increases
D. (F) CBF increases
E. (T)

57. A. (T)
B. (F) travels in the posterior columns
C. (F) travels in the posterior columns
D. (T)
E. (F) travels in the posterior columns

58. A. (T)
B. (F) these are cholinergic
C. (F) all autonomic preganglionic neurons are cholinergic
D. (F)
E. (F) these are cholinergic

59. A. (T)
B. (F) contraction
C. (T) for near vision
D. (F) contraction
E. (F) erection

60. A. (T)
B. (T)
C. (F) this inhibits gastrin secretion
D. (F) this hormone inhibits gastrin secretion
E. (T)

61. A. (F)
B. (F)
C. (T)

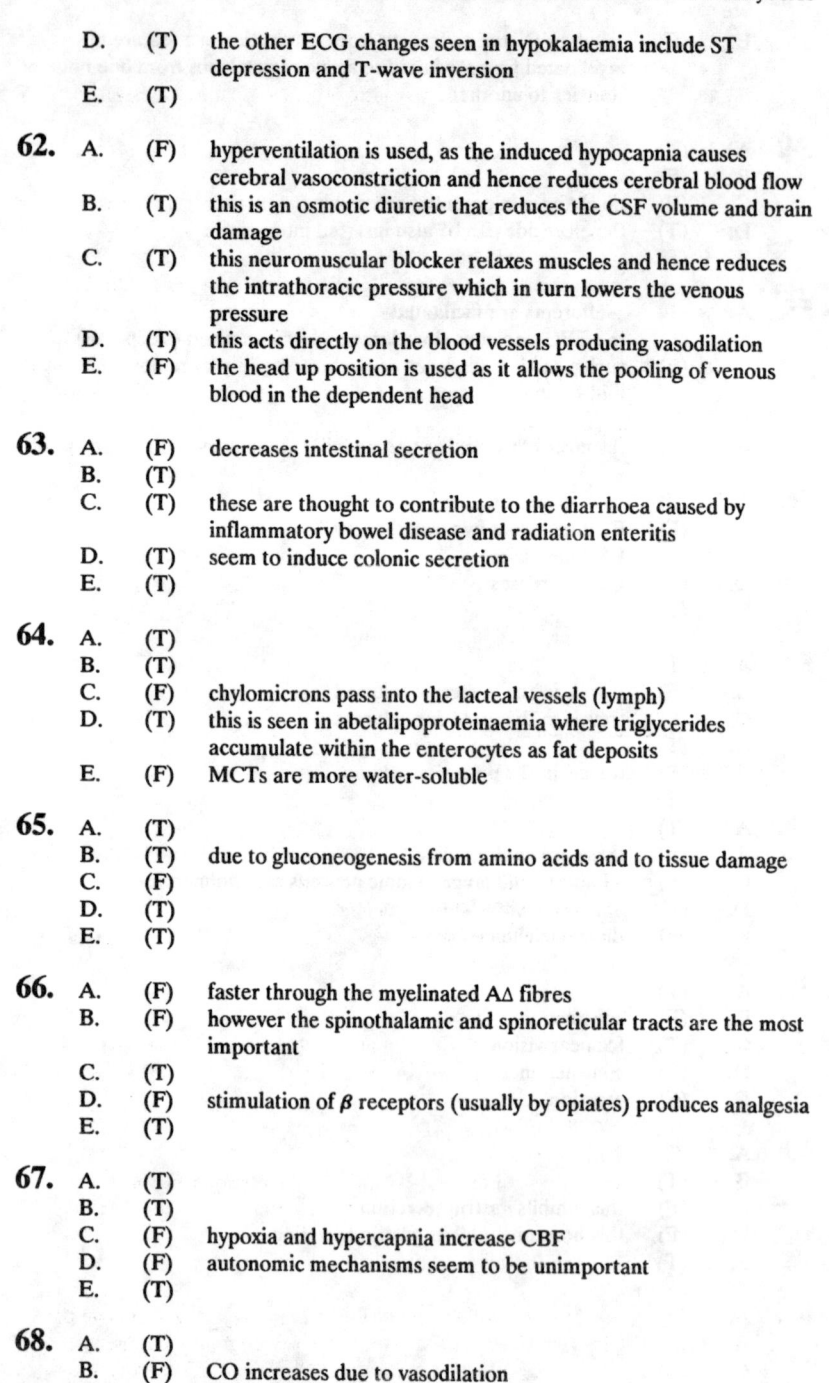

	D.	(T)	the other ECG changes seen in hypokalaemia include ST depression and T-wave inversion
	E.	(T)	
62.	A.	(F)	hyperventilation is used, as the induced hypocapnia causes cerebral vasoconstriction and hence reduces cerebral blood flow
	B.	(T)	this is an osmotic diuretic that reduces the CSF volume and brain damage
	C.	(T)	this neuromuscular blocker relaxes muscles and hence reduces the intrathoracic pressure which in turn lowers the venous pressure
	D.	(T)	this acts directly on the blood vessels producing vasodilation
	E.	(F)	the head up position is used as it allows the pooling of venous blood in the dependent head
63.	A.	(F)	decreases intestinal secretion
	B.	(T)	
	C.	(T)	these are thought to contribute to the diarrhoea caused by inflammatory bowel disease and radiation enteritis
	D.	(T)	seem to induce colonic secretion
	E.	(T)	
64.	A.	(T)	
	B.	(T)	
	C.	(F)	chylomicrons pass into the lacteal vessels (lymph)
	D.	(T)	this is seen in abetalipoproteinaemia where triglycerides accumulate within the enterocytes as fat deposits
	E.	(F)	MCTs are more water-soluble
65.	A.	(T)	
	B.	(T)	due to gluconeogenesis from amino acids and to tissue damage
	C.	(F)	
	D.	(T)	
	E.	(T)	
66.	A.	(F)	faster through the myelinated AΔ fibres
	B.	(F)	however the spinothalamic and spinoreticular tracts are the most important
	C.	(T)	
	D.	(F)	stimulation of β receptors (usually by opiates) produces analgesia
	E.	(T)	
67.	A.	(T)	
	B.	(T)	
	C.	(F)	hypoxia and hypercapnia increase CBF
	D.	(F)	autonomic mechanisms seem to be unimportant
	E.	(T)	
68.	A.	(T)	
	B.	(F)	CO increases due to vasodilation

	C.	(T)	
	D.	(F)	CO usually increases
	E.	(T)	this drug blocks the parasympathetic output to the heart
69.	A.	(F)	
	B.	(T)	
	C.	(F)	Na$^+$ absorption is not influenced by intraluminal glucose or amino acids (See Figure 14)
	D.	(T)	aldosterone increases rate of absorption
	E.	(T)	this accounts for about 15% of basal energy requirement

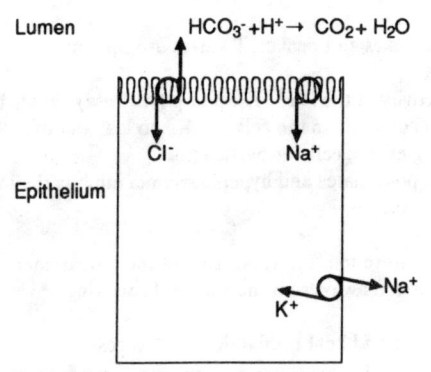

Transcellular absorption and secretion

Figure 14

70.	A.	(T)	by coating red blood cells. Therefore blood should be taken for cross-matching before dextran administration
	B.	(F)	this is a feature of dextran 40
	C.	(F)	the half-life is about 16 days
	D.	(F)	allergic reactions are rare (<0.1% of cases)
	E.	(T)	
71.	A.	(T)	due to increased total peripheral resistance and to a direct negative inotropic effect on the heart
	B.	(T)	vasopressor action
	C.	(F)	ACTH release is increased
	D.	(T)	with water
	E.	(F)	the release of factor VIII and von Willebrand's factor is increased thus contributing to haemostasis
72.	A.	(F)	the secretion is pulsatile
	B.	(T)	
	C.	(T)	e.g. buserelin or goserelin. These analogues down-regulate the pituitary receptors to decrease the secretion of LH. They maybe combined with other drugs e.g. cyproterone which block the

			action of testosterone
	D.	(T)	e.g. induction of ovulation in the female, azoospermia in the male
	E.	(F)	LH response is greater in the luteal phase
73.	A.	(T)	
	B.	(T)	therefore antiemetics acting at CTZ don't need to penetrate this barrier to be effective
	C.	(F)	$5HT_3$ antagonists may be effective
	D.	(T)	
	E.	(F)	H_1-receptors have been identified in the vomiting centre
74.	A.	(T)	
	B.	(T)	
	C.	(F)	wide QRS complexes and peaked T-waves are seen in hyperkalaemia
	D.	(T)	the reduced activity of the Na^+-K^+ pump (ATPase) causes Na^+ and water to accumulate in the cell and K^+ to leak out of it. The cellular swelling causes cellular dysfunction
	E.	(F)	hypocalcaemia potentiates and hypercalcaemia inhibits the local anaesthetic action
75.	A.	(T)	i.e. body temperature tends to reach that of the environment
	B.	(T)	blood flow diversion away from the skin and shivering are inhibited
	C.	(F)	the metabolic rate and heat production are depressed
	D.	(T)	
	E.	(F)	hyperkalaemia and acidosis are characteristic
76.	A.	(F)	in the form of crystalline amino acids
	B.	(F)	
	C.	(F)	these amino acids may precipitate and worsen hepatic encephalopathy. Branched chain amino acids are recommended
	D.	(T)	if infusion is given too rapidly. The solution is hypertonic
	E.	(T)	trace elements should be given daily. Zinc requirements are increased in patients with bowel fistulae

Clinical Pharmacology

1. **Heparin**

    A. may cause thrombocytopenia
    B. anticoagulation is best monitored by measuring INR
    C. is antagonized by protamin sulphate
    D. has a longer duration of action when administered subcutaneously rather than intravenously
    E. is usually given as 5000 units subcutaneously twice daily to treat an established DVT

2. **Warfarin**

    A. anticoagulation is effective 24 hours after the first dose
    B. is well absorbed from the alimentary tract
    C. has a half-life of about 36 hours
    D. action is terminated mainly by renal excretion
    E. metabolism by the liver is induced by cimetidine

3. **Frusemide**

    A. inhibits active chloride re-absorption in the thick segment of ascending loop of Henle
    B. decreases calcium and magnesium excretion in urine
    C. to be preferred to thiazides in a patient with a GFR of 12 ml/min
    D. is safely given in combination with gentamicin
    E. is antagonized by indomethacin

4. **The following statements refer to insulin**

    A. most insulin-dependent diabetics require about 70 units per day
    B. soluble insulin (acid or neutral) is the only type suitable for intravenous administration
    C. the crystalline form of insulin zinc suspension has an intermediate duration of action (12–16 hours)
    D. insulin requirements increase in diabetic patients undergoing major surgery
    E. insulin requirements decrease in bacterial septicaemia as bacteria utilize blood glucose

5. The following statements refer to oral hypoglycaemics

   A. metformin is effective in pancreatectomized animals
   B. sulphonylureas stimulate isolated islets of Langerhans to release insulin *in vitro*
   C. chlorpropamide is the oral hypoglycaemic of choice in a maturity-onset diabetic with heart failure
   D. tolbutamide is to be preferred to chlorpropamide in an elderly patient with renal failure
   E. lactic acidosis is a recognized side effect of phenformin and metformin administration

6. Metronidazole

   A. inhibits alcohol and aldehyde dehydrogenase
   B. impairs the formation of nucleic acids in anaerobic micro-organisms
   C. has been shown to be carcinogenic in humans
   D. has peripheral neuropathy as a recognized side effect
   E. is effective against *Entamoeba histolytica*

7. With respect to benzodiazepines

   A. diazepam has a longer plasma half-time than temazepam
   B. temazepam has active metabolites
   C. benzodiazepines antagonize gamma-aminobutyric acid (GABA) in the brain
   D. benzodiazepines prolong the duration of total sleep
   E. benzodiazepines have anticonvulsant and muscle relaxant actions

8. Non-steroidal anti-inflammatory drugs (NSAIDs)

   A. inhibit the enzyme cyclo-oxygenase which converts arachidonic acid to cyclic endoperoxides
   B. may cause the closure of a patent ductus arteriosus after birth
   C. reduce gastric acid secretion
   D. potentiate the antihypertensive effect of β-blockers
   E. can inhibit thromboxane synthetase in platelets

9. Morphine

   A. stimulates the chemoreceptor trigger zone
   B. causes spasm of the sphincter of Oddi
   C. inhibits the third cranial nerve nucleus
   D. suppresses anti-diuretic hormone (ADH) secretion
   E. reduces the tone in the gut wall

CLINICAL PHARMACOLOGY

10. Morphine

- A. undergoes negligible first pass metabolism when given orally
- B. is mainly eliminated unchanged by the kidneys
- C. has a duration of useful analgesia of about 5 hours
- D. is dangerous to use in a patient with emphysema
- E. may be beneficial in a patient with left ventricular failure

11. Omeprazole

- A. inhibits the H^+, K^+-ATPase in the secretory canaliculi of the oxyntic cell
- B. has a short duration of action (about 3 hours)
- C. can stimulate excessive gastrin release causing hypergastrinaemia
- D. has been shown to produce carcinoid tumours in rats when used in high doses
- E. induces the microsomal enzymes of the liver

12. With respect to aminoglycosides

- A. kanamycin is the most effective against *Ps. aeruginosa*
- B. the topical use of neomycin has not been shown to cause VIII cranial nerve palsy
- C. aminoglycosides exert their bacterial effect by binding to the microbial ribosomes
- D. gentamicin is active against anaerobes
- E. gentamicin is the drug of choice for Gram-negative septicaemia

13. Cefuroxime

- A. is a third generation cephalosporin
- B. possesses a B-lactam ring which binds to bacterial enzymes which are necessary for the synthesis of the cell wall
- C. shows cross sensitivity with penicillins
- D. has poor penetration into the CSF
- E. is a useful prophylactic antibiotic in cholecystectomy

14. Cimetidine

- A. reduces the volume and the hydrogen ion concentration of gastric juice
- B. blocks androgen receptors
- C. inhibits the proton pump in the parietal cells
- D. is mainly excreted unchanged in urine
- E. blocks both H_1 and H_2 receptors

15. Ranitidine

A. does not inhibit gastric acid secretion provoked by acetylcholine
B. has a similar half-life to cimetidine
C. is excreted mainly unchanged by the kidneys
D. blocks androgen receptors
E. inhibits hepatic drug oxidizing enzymes

16. The clinical uses of cimetidine include

A. chronic pancreatic insufficiency
B. Zollinger–Ellison syndrome
C. reflux oesophagitis
D. stomal ulceration
E. bradycardia

17. Carbenoxolone

A. enhances gastric mucosal resistance
B. reduces back diffusion of H^+ ion from the lumen into the mucosa
C. antagonizes aldosterone
D. is excreted mainly unchanged in urine
E. is preferred to ranitidine when treating a gastric ulcer in the elderly

18. The drugs used in management of reflux oesophagitis include

A. anatacids combined with alginic acid
B. chlorpromazine
C. H_1 receptor blockers
D. metoclopramide
E. atropine

19. Figure 15 shows the various sites of tubular reabsorption of sodium and water along the nephron

with respect to the action of diuretics

A. zone III is the primary site of action of mannitol
B. frusemide inhibits chloride reabsorption (and Na^+) in zones II and III
C. amiloride acting on zone IV promotes the loss of H^+ in urine
D. thiazide (acting on zone III) promotes K^+ loss in urine in zone IV
E. acetazolamide acting on zones I and IV produces acidic urine

CLINICAL PHARMACOLOGY 77

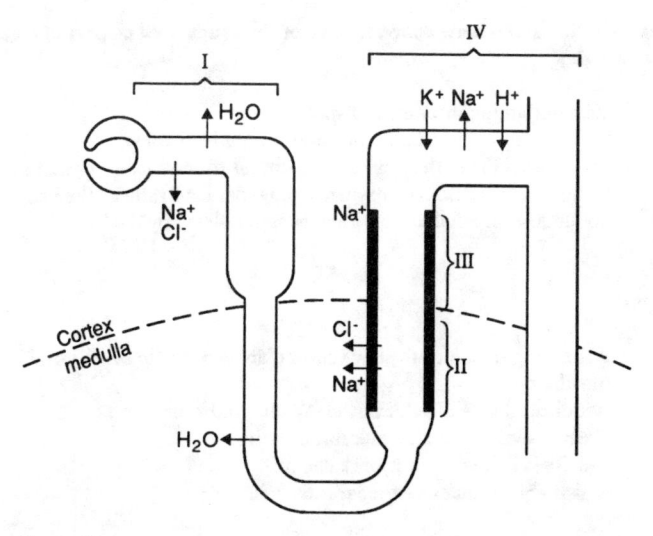

Figure 15

20. The following drugs are cleared mainly by hepatic mechanisms

　　A. heparin
　　B. warfarin
　　C. cyclosporin
　　D. acyclovir
　　E. vancomycin

21. Lignocaine when used as a local anaesthetic (LA)

　　A. inhibits the rapid inflow of Na^+ into excitable cells
　　B. reduces the resting transmembrane potential of excitable cells
　　C. is a more active LA if injected into an inflamed area
　　D. may cause cardiac arrest
　　E. has a local anaesthetic action lasting for about 1 hour (1% lignocaine)

22. The following statements refer to some drugs used in the treatment of cancer

　　A. 6-mercaptopurine is a sulphur analogue of adenine
　　B. cisplatin is the most effective single agent against testicular teratomas
　　C. tamoxifen has a plasma half-life of 6 hours
　　D. tamoxifen has a low toxicity
　　E. cyclophosphamide is an active cytotoxic alkylating agent which is converted by liver microsomal enzymes to inactive metabolites

23. The following statements concern some of the drugs used as part of a general anaesthetic

   A. suxamethonium may cause hypokalaemia
   B. thiopentone is absolutely contra-indicated in porphyria
   C. ketamine reduces the sympathetic output to the cardiovascular system
   D. isoflurane increases the oxygen supply–demand ratio of the brain
   E. about 20% of inhaled isoflurane is metabolized by the liver

24. Digoxin

   A. is the drug of choice to slow ventricular response in acute atrial fibrillation
   B. is indicated in Wolf–Parkinson–White syndrome
   C. plasma levels should be measured routinely
   D. toxicity is increased in hyperkalaemia
   E. is available as an elixir preparation

Answers

1.
   A. (T)
   B. (F) the KCCT is used to monitor heparin anticoagulation
   C. (T)
   D. (T)
   E. (F) this regimen is suitable for the prophylaxis of DVT in high risk patients

2.
   A. (F) 72 hours after the first dose. This is because the clotting factors already present in the circulation need to be eliminated
   B. (T) this is the main advantage over heparin
   C. (F) T½ is about 36 hours
   D. (F) by hepatic metabolism
   E. (F) cimetidine inhibits the enzyme system which metabolizes warfarin

3.
   A. (T)
   B. (F) increases Ca^{2+} and Mg^{2+} urinary excretion
   C. (T) frusemide has a higher efficacy in the cases of low GFR than other diuretics
   D. (F) gentamicin renal excretion may be reduced leading to nephrotoxicity and ototoxicity
   E. (T)

4.
   A. (F) most require about 40 units per day
   B. (T)
   C. (F) this is a long acting insulin with activity lasting 30–36 hours

CLINICAL PHARMACOLOGY

	D.	(T)	
	E.	(F)	the requirements usually increase in infections (by up to one third of the usual dose)
5.	A.	(T)	does not seem to rely on B-cells for its actions
	B.	(T)	
	C.	(F)	it has an anti-diuretic effect (ADH-like) which causes water retention and dilutional hyponatraemia
	D.	(T)	tolbutamide which has a shorter duration of action is mainly metabolized in the liver, whereas chlorpropamide is mainly excreted unchanged in urine
	E.	(T)	
6.	A.	(T)	causing a disulphiram-like action
	B.	(T)	it is converted to a compound which binds to DNA
	C.	(F)	large doses have been shown to be carcinogenic in rodents, but no study has shown carcinogenicity in humans
	D.	(T)	
	E.	(T)	
7.	A.	(T)	$T_{1/2}$ (diazepam) = 30 hours; $T_{1/2}$ (temazepam) = 10 hours
	B.	(F)	
	C.	(F)	they enhance the effects of GABA
	D.	(T)	
	E.	(T)	
8.	A.	(T)	thus inhibiting prostaglandin synthesis
	B.	(T)	this is a recognized therapeutic measure
	C.	(F)	NSAIDs commonly damage intestinal and gastric mucosa. This in effect is due to inhibition of prostaglandin synthesis. The latter inhibit gastric acid secretion and exert a cytoprotective effect
	D.	(F)	NSAIDs antagonize the antihypertensive effect of β-blockers by causing Na^+ and water retention due to inhibition of renal prostaglandins
	E.	(T)	this is the basis for their use against occlusive vascular disease
9.	A.	(T)	causing nausea and vomiting
	B.	(T)	pethidine is to be preferred to morphine in biliary colic
	C.	(F)	morphine stimulates this nucleus causing miosis
	D.	(F)	it stimulates ADH release
	E.	(F)	morphine stimulates the smooth muscle of the intestine which becomes in a state of tonic contraction leading to constipation. Peristalsis is inhibited
10.	A.	(F)	extensive first-pass metabolism occurs
	B.	(F)	morphine undergoes both hepatic and renal metabolism, and only 10% of it is excreted unchanged in urine
	C.	(T)	$T_{1/2}$ is 2–4 hours
	D.	(T)	it decreases the response to arterial PCO_2
	E.	(T)	venodilation relieves the pre-load of the heart

11.
A. (T)
B. (F) has a long-lasting action (>12 hours)
C. (T) by decreasing the negative feedback of HCl
D. (T)
E. (F) the microsomal enzymes may be inhibited

12.
A. (F) it has little efficacy against this organism. Tobramycin is to be preferred
B. (F) the absorption can be sufficient to cause this side effect
C. (T)
D. (F)
E. (T)

13.
A. (F) a second generation cephalosporin
B. (T)
C. (T)
D. (F) has good penetration, therefore it is of value in the treatment of bacterial meningitis
E. (T)

14.
A. (T)
B. (T) causing gynaecomastia and impotence
C. (F)
D. (T)
E. (F) blocks H_2 receptors only

15.
A. (F)
B. (T)
C. (T)
D. (F) this explains why it does not cause gynaecomastia or impotence (cf. cimetidine)
E. (F) (cf. cimetidine)

16.
A. (T)
B. (T)
C. (T)
D. (T)
E. (F) this is a recognized side effect of the drug

17.
A. (T)
B. (T)
C. (F) it has an aldosterone-like action
D. (F) it is excreted mainly unchanged in the bile
E. (F) from C, it is clear that carbenoxolone may lead to hypertension and heart failure due to Na^+ retention. It should therefore be avoided in the elderly

18.
A. (T)
B. (F)
C. (F)

CLINICAL PHARMACOLOGY

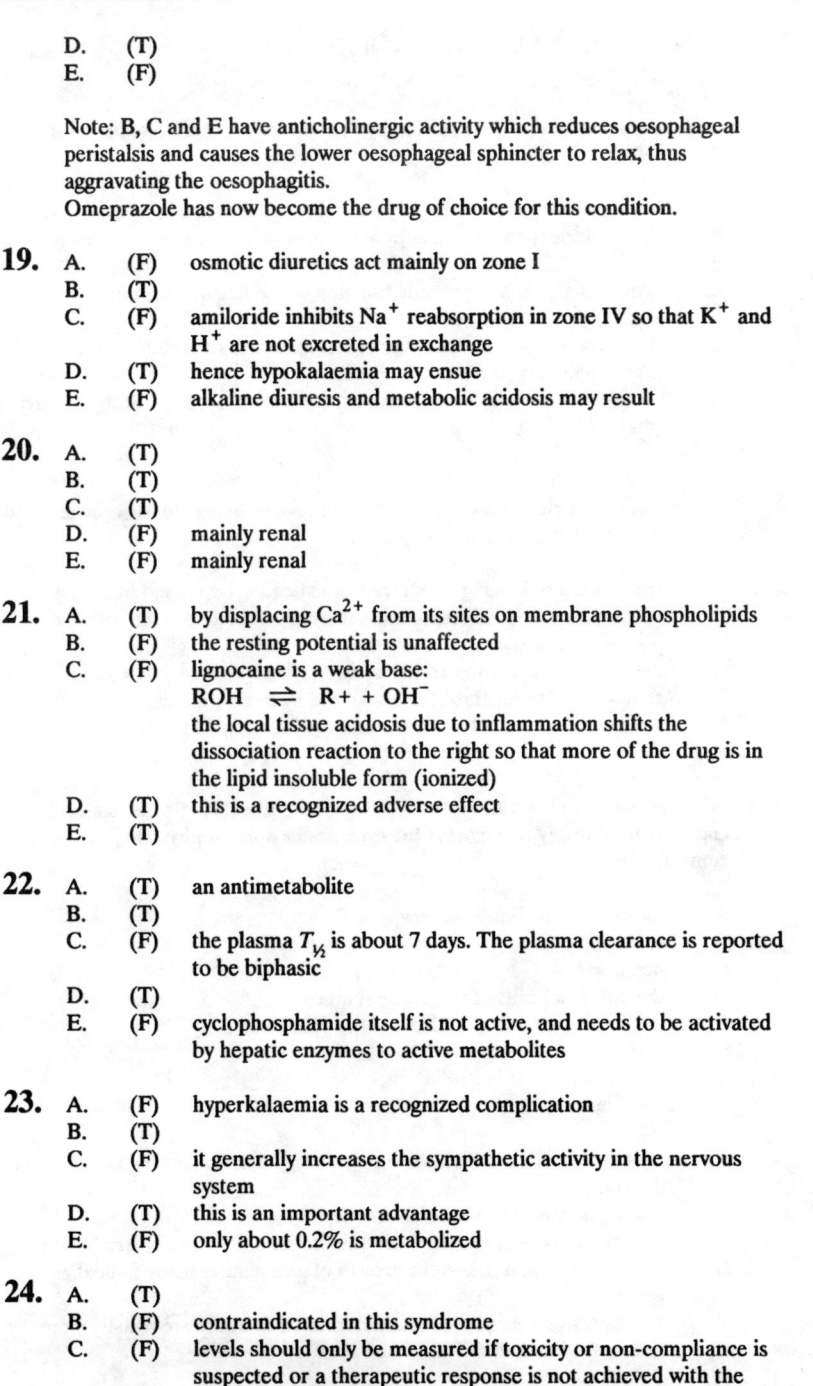

    D. (T)
    E. (F)

Note: B, C and E have anticholinergic activity which reduces oesophageal peristalsis and causes the lower oesophageal sphincter to relax, thus aggravating the oesophagitis.
Omeprazole has now become the drug of choice for this condition.

19.
- A. (F) osmotic diuretics act mainly on zone I
- B. (T)
- C. (F) amiloride inhibits Na^+ reabsorption in zone IV so that K^+ and H^+ are not excreted in exchange
- D. (T) hence hypokalaemia may ensue
- E. (F) alkaline diuresis and metabolic acidosis may result

20.
- A. (T)
- B. (T)
- C. (T)
- D. (F) mainly renal
- E. (F) mainly renal

21.
- A. (T) by displacing Ca^{2+} from its sites on membrane phospholipids
- B. (F) the resting potential is unaffected
- C. (F) lignocaine is a weak base:
  $$ROH \rightleftharpoons R+ + OH^-$$
  the local tissue acidosis due to inflammation shifts the dissociation reaction to the right so that more of the drug is in the lipid insoluble form (ionized)
- D. (T) this is a recognized adverse effect
- E. (T)

22.
- A. (T) an antimetabolite
- B. (T)
- C. (F) the plasma $T_{½}$ is about 7 days. The plasma clearance is reported to be biphasic
- D. (T)
- E. (F) cyclophosphamide itself is not active, and needs to be activated by hepatic enzymes to active metabolites

23.
- A. (F) hyperkalaemia is a recognized complication
- B. (T)
- C. (F) it generally increases the sympathetic activity in the nervous system
- D. (T) this is an important advantage
- E. (F) only about 0.2% is metabolized

24.
- A. (T)
- B. (F) contraindicated in this syndrome
- C. (F) levels should only be measured if toxicity or non-compliance is suspected or a therapeutic response is not achieved with the expected dose
- D. (F) hypokalaemia increases toxicity
- E. (T)

General and Systemic Pathology

1. Considering a small wound healing by first intention which has been sutured by monofilament nylon (assuming no complications)

    A. monocytes help to clean away the debris by phagocytes
    B. the epidermal and dermal epithelia grow downwards along the suture track
    C. fibroblasts have a contractile function which helps to produce a small scar
    D. the early removal of sutures does not influence the extent of the granulomatosis response
    E. the wound site is as vascular during the fourth week as during the first week of healing

2. When suturing a clean incision with the skin edges being closely apposed and considering that there are no complications

    A. the process of healing is referred to as healing by second intention
    B. usually there is no acute inflammatory reaction associated with the process of healing
    C. new collagen is demonstrable in the wound by the second day
    D. reticulin is demonstrable in the wound by the third day
    E. a continuous layer of epidermis usually forms in 48 hours

3. With respect to regeneration, the following cells are classified as labile (i.e. continue to multiply throughout life even under normal physiological conditions)

    A. the cells of the bone marrow
    B. cerebral neurons
    C. hepatocytes
    D. the epithelial cells of the tracheal mucosa
    E. the squamous cell epithelium of the epidermis

4. Ionizing radiation

    A. cells are usually most sensitive to ionizing radiation during G1 phase of the cell cycle
    B. mitosis may occur in irradiated cells
    C. hypoxia makes cells particularly vulnerable to damage by irradiation
    D. ionizing radiation delays the growth of granulation tissue in healing wounds
    E. within any tumour group, undifferentiated tumours are usually more radiosensitive than differentiated ones

5. Considering the genetic basis of disease

A. in autosomal dominant inheritance, the abnormal gene may be situated on a sex chromosome
B. in autosomal dominant inheritance, the disease is always transmitted by an affected parent
C. in autosomal recessive inheritance, if two carrier parents marry there is 25% chance of each child being affected
D. the genes coding for the human leukocyte antigen (HLA) are located on the long arm of chromosome 6
E. Graves' disease is associated with HLA types DR3 and B8

6. The following statements are correct

A. autolytic changes in the nucleus are pathognomonic of necrosis
B. necrotic tissue usually provokes an acute inflammatory reaction in the surrounding tissue
C. gangrene is synonymous with necrosis
D. the blood vessels in an acutely inflamed part usually show progressive vasodilation from the time of injury
E. apoptosis is usually associated with an inflammatory response

7. Considering cell response to injury

A. in hypoxic cells K^+ is retained in the cells and Na^+ escapes from them
B. hypoxia does not lead to the formation of powerful oxidants in cells due to lack of oxygen
C. in hydropic degeneration the cells are typically dehydrated
D. fatty change is a recognized cell response to damage by poisons or hypoxia
E. a free radical is a molecule that contains an odd number of electrons

8. With respect to disorder of cell growth

A. the stimulus to hypertrophy is usually hormonal
B. atrophy may be caused by ionizing radiation
C. hypocalcaemia may cause hyperplasia of the thyroid gland
D. achondroplasia does not affect membrane bones
E. in metaplasia there is a change of one type of differentiated cell to another type of undifferentiated cell

9. **Wound healing**

   A. when collagen is synthesized hydroxyproline and hydroxylysine are incorporated directly into the collagen molecule
   B. collagen lysis is increased in infected wounds
   C. the wound weakens in scurvy due to increased activity of collagenase
   D. when using absorbable sutures, the wound strength progressively increases to maximum from the time of suturing
   E. the inflammatory response to suture insertion is greater for monofilamentous nylon than for catgut

10. **With respect to cancer**

    A. as the tumour becomes larger the rate of growth slows down
    B. there is evidence that natural killer cells (NK) are involved in the destruction of tumour cells
    C. malignant cells show loss of both density dependent inhibition of growth and contact inhibition
    D. protease activity is characteristically reduced in malignant cells
    E. polyposis coli, which is pre-cancerous, is inherited in an autosomal recessive fashion

11. **With respect to chemical carcinogens**

    A. all carcinogens require further metabolism to become carcinogenic
    B. Ames assay is a useful screening test for potential carcinogens
    C. most carcinogens are initiating agents only, i.e. require promoters to cause tumours
    D. cytochrome P-448 (monooxygenase) is involved in the conversion of procarcinogens into ultimate carcinogens
    E. the DNA damage caused by covalent interaction with the carcinogen cannot be repaired

12. **Oncogenes**

    A. are genes capable of causing cancer
    B. have been isolated from about 50% of human cancers
    C. about 50% of the products of the known viral oncogenes are protein kinases
    D. may uncouple the intranuclear mechanisms involved in growth control from the need for an external stimulus
    E. growth suppressor genes are a good example of oncogenes

GENERAL AND SYSTEMIC PATHOLOGY

13. With respect to fracture healing

   A. the cells of the deeper layer of the periosteum have osteogenic potential
   B. the pH of the uniting fracture starts decreasing after about 10 days
   C. the bone ends show osteoporosis in the early stages of fracture healing
   D. woven bone formation is more likely to occur than cartilage formation whenever there is mobilization
   E. globules of fat may enter disrupted vascular spaces and become embolic

14. Carcinoma of the bladder urothelium

   A. β-naphthylamine itself is not carcinogenic
   B. grade 1 carcinoma has a better prognosis than grade 3 carcinoma
   C. direct spread through Denonvillier's fascia is common
   D. if it is thought that the tumour penetrated through the bladder wall but has not reached the pelvic wall, the tumour will be stage T2 according to TNM classification
   E. squamous cell carcinoma is more radiosensitive than adenocarcinoma

15. The following are commoner in Crohn's disease than in ulcerative colitis

   A. crypt abscesses in the bowel mucosa
   B. pseudopolyps in the bowel lumen
   C. the development of carcinoma as a complication
   D. bowel obstruction as a complication
   E. involvement of the submucosa and deeper layers

16. Osteosarcoma

   A. is more likely to spread (from the diaphysis) to the epiphyses in children than in adults
   B. the lungs are the commonest sites for distant metastases
   C. the neoplastic cells may produce cartilage and fibrous tissue
   D. shows no sex predilection
   E. the juxtacortical variety has a better prognosis than the medullary variety

17. Hyperplasia

   A. enlargement of an organ due to inflammation is an example of hyperplasia
   B. hyperplasia due to a specific stimulus usually persists even if the stimulus is withdrawn
   C. there is epithelial hyperplasia in benign prostatic enlargement
   D. is seen in the myocardium in systemic hypertension
   E. parathyroid glands may undergo hyperplasia in chronic renal failure

18. Acute haemorrhagic pancreatitis

A. trauma is a recognized aetiological factor
B. the foci of fat necrosis appear as small black nodules
C. elastase and trypsin play a role in the pathogenesis of haemorrhage and thrombosis
D. the contents of a pseudocyst (which may complicate the condition) are confined by an epithelial capsule
E. hypocalcaemia ensues due to the consumption of calcium as it combines with amino acids

19. Breast cancer

A. there is an approximately twenty-fold increase in breast cancer among first degree relatives of women who have had breast cancer
B. the incidence of breast cancer shows geographical variation
C. intraductal carcinoma is more likely to produce a palpable breast mass than *in situ* lobular carcinoma
D. in *in situ* lobular carcinoma, the terminal ducts are distended and their central lumens are obliterated by tumour cells
E. intraductal carcinoma produces nipple discharge in most cases

20. Invasive breast cancer

A. the lobular histological type has the most favourable prognosis
B. there is a good correlation between the ten-years survival rate and the number of axillary lymph nodes involved at diagnosis
C. the risk of development of contralateral breast cancer is greatest in the medullary histological type
D. the colloid carcinoma is characterized by mucus produced by tumour cells
E. there is an inverse relationship between the diameter of the tumour and the 5-year survival rate

21. Figure 16 represents different phases of the cell cycle

The following statements are correct

A. cells are most sensitive to ionizing radiation during the S-phase
B. DNA synthesis is confined to the S-phase
C. during G1 phase, the cells are metabolically inactive
D. the total duration of the cell cycle in normal tissues is constant
E. the cells of solid tumours in humans all proceed through the cell cycle in the same phase

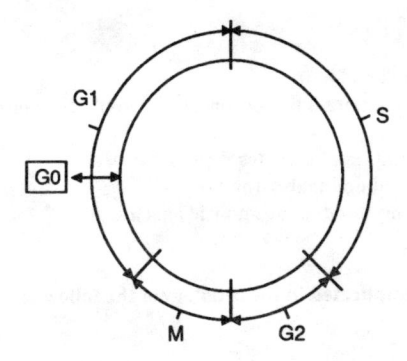

Figure 16

22. Irrigating the bladder with glycine solution when performing TURP may lead to

- A. increased total body sodium
- B. increased osmolality of the plasma
- C. hyponatraemia
- D. cerebral oedema
- E. hypertension and bradycardia

23. The following are recognized causes of mycotic aneurysms

- A. *Mycobacterium tuberculosis*
- B. *Staphylococcus aureus*
- C. Marfan's syndrome
- D. *Streptococcus viridans*
- E. *Trichophyton rubrum*

24. The carcinoid syndrome

- A. occurs once 5-hydroxytryptamine is secreted into the portal vein by a carcinoid tumour
- B. most commonly follows carcinoid tumours of the colon
- C. affects the left side of the heart more frequently than the right side
- D. may cause bronchospasm
- E. is associated with increased urinary excretion of 5-hydroxyindoleacetic acid (5HIAA)

25. Cholesterol gallstones

A. are usually multiple, small and hard
B. do not form in bile that contains a molar concentration of cholesterol of about 30%
C. are a recognized complication of diabetes mellitus
D. may be visible on a plain abdominal X-ray
E. commonly develop in long-standing haemolytic anaemias

26. Epstein–Barr virus has been implicated in the aetiology of the following cancers in man

A. carcinoma of the cervix
B. Hodgkin's lymphoma
C. cerebral astrocytoma
D. Burkitt's lymphoma
E. nasopharyngeal carcinoma

27. The following statements are correct

A. faecoliths are found in more than 50% of acutely inflamed appendices
B. villous adenoma is a hamartoma
C. tubular and villous adenomas are precancerous
D. the bronchus is the commonest site for carcinoid tumour
E. gastric ulcers most commonly occur on the greater curvature of the stomach

28. Carcinoma of the stomach

A. the incidence is 10 times higher in individuals with chronic atrophic gastritis
B. linitis plastica has a better prognosis than polypoid carcinoma
C. in malignant gastric ulcers the mucosal folds usually converge on ulcer without interruption
D. Krukenberg tumour is characterized by signet ring neoplastic cells with abundant fibrous tissue stroma
E. metastasis to the left supraclavicular lymph nodes occurs through the thoracic duct

29. Carcinoma of the thyroid

A. papillary carcinoma carries the most favourable prognosis
B. follicular carcinoma is characterized by psammoma bodies
C. follicular carcinomas commonly metastasizes to regional lymph nodes
D. medullary carcinoma may be inherited in an autosomal dominant fashion
E. anaplastic carcinoma often secretes calcitonin

30. Carcinoma of the colon and rectum

A. approximately 75% of carcinomas occur in the rectum and sigmoid colon
B. tumours in the right colon are more likely to produce obstruction than those in the left colon
C. signet ring cells may be seen on microscopy
D. Duke used the term 'stage D' for carcinoma with distant metastases
E. in Duke's stage D the regional lymph nodes are involved

31. The following skin lesions have a malignant potential

A. dermoid cyst
B. cavernous haemangioma
C. Bowen's disease
D. intradermal naevus
E. erythroplasia of Queyrat

32. The following favours a good prognosis in melanoma

A. male sex
B. a low Breslow thickness
C. amelanosis
D. involvement of trunk
E. regional lymphadenopathy

33. Cerebral aneurysms

A. are commoner in males
B. are more likely to rupture when they are giant
C. usually rupture at the fundus of the aneurysm
D. may present with a III nerve palsy
E. usually present with the features of subarachnoid haemorrhage

34. The following refer to peripheral nerve injuries

A. recovery from neuropraxia is usually complete in 7 weeks
B. in axonotmesis there is disruption of the continuity of the nerve sheath
C. primary suturing of a divided nerve should be performed immediately even if the wound is contaminated
D. functional recovery from neurotmesis is usually complete if time is allowed for regeneration
E. the rate of regeneration in axonotmesis is about 1 mm per day

35. The causes of communicating hydrocephalus include

A. Arnold–Chiari malformation
B. TB meningitis
C. subarachnoid haemorrhage
D. head injury
E. stenosis of the aqueduct of Sylvius

36. The consequences of chronic liver disease include

A. hypergammaglobulinaemia
B. hypoalbuminaemia
C. encephalopathy
D. low plasma levels of von Willebrand's factor
E. hypercholesterolaemia

37. Fat embolus

A. may arise from plasma lipids
B. usually occurs about 10 days after major fractures
C. passes through the pulmonary filter to the cerebral circulation in most cases
D. is associated with increased plasma lipase levels in about 50% of cases
E. commonly causes pyoderma gangrenosum

38. The following are recognized causes of amyloidosis

A. Hodgkin's disease
B. extradural haematoma secondary to head injury
C. inflammatory bowel disease
D. chronic suppurative infections
E. hiatus hernia

39. The following factors impair wound healing

A. zinc deficiency
B. excessive tension in the sutures
C. uraemia
D. rheumatoid arthritis
E. ultraviolet light

Answers

1. A. (T)
   B. (T) to form an incomplete tube of epithelium around the whole suture
   C. (T)
   D. (F) the early removal decreases the extent of granulation
   E. (F) the vascular elements decrease with time until the scar becomes almost avascular

2. A. (F) healing by first intention
   B. (F) a mild acute inflammatory reaction usually occurs within 24 hours
   C. (F) by the fifth day
   D. (T)
   E. (T)

3. A. (T)
   B. (F) these are 'permanent' cells, i.e. they lose their ability to proliferate around the time of birth
   C. (F) these are 'stable' cells
   D. (T)
   E. (T)

4. A. (F) maximum radiosensitivity occurs during mitosis. During G1 phase cells are relatively radioresistant
   B. (T)
   C. (F) hypoxia provides a protective effect against radiation, e.g. the centre of a malignant mass is relatively protected by hypoxia
   D. (T)
   E. (T)

5. A. (F) the gene is located on autosomes
   B. (F) an example of exception is neurofibromatosis where there is a high spontaneous mutation rate
   C. (T)
   D. (F) on the short arm of chromosome 6
   E. (T)

6. A. (T)
   B. (T)
   C. (F) gangrene is necrosis with superadded putrefaction
   D. (F) there is initial vasoconstriction, probably due to direct mechanical stimulation
   E. (F) there is no inflammatory reaction in apoptosis

7. A. (F) the activity of the sodium pump is reduced, leading to accumulation of Na^+ in the cell and escape of K^+ out of the cell
   B. (F) the formation of powerful oxidants (e.g. O_2^- free radical) contributes to cell damage

	C.	(F)	the cells are waterlogged
	D.	(T)	
	E.	(T)	e.g. O_2^- which is highly active
8.	A.	(F)	usually mechanical
	B.	(T)	post-irradiation atrophy
	C.	(F)	
	D.	(T)	cartilage bones are affected
	E.	(F)	the change is from one type of differentiated cell to another type of differentiated cell
9.	A.	(F)	lysine and proline are incorporated into the protocollagen molecule which is acted upon by protocollagen hydroxylase
	B.	(T)	
	C.	(F)	ascorbic acid is required for protocollagen hydroxylase. The wound weakness is due to impaired collagen synthesis
	D.	(F)	See Figure 17

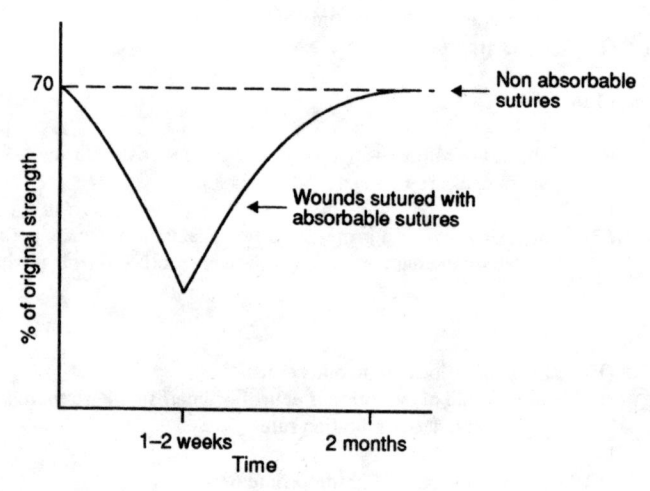

Figure 17

	E.	(F)	there is less tissue reaction with synthetic monofilamentous sutures
10.	A.	(T)	
	B.	(T)	
	C.	(T)	
	D.	(F)	the protease activity is increased in malignant cells
	E.	(F)	autosomal dominant inheritance
11.	A.	(F)	some are direct carcinogens
	B.	(T)	the test looks for the ability of compounds to produce a mutation in one of the genes of *Salmonella typhimurium*
	C.	(F)	most carcinogens are both initiating agents and promotors

GENERAL AND SYSTEMIC PATHOLOGY

    D.   (T)
    E.   (F)   the damage can be repaired by the repair systems. The persistence of certain types of damage for a long time may be responsible for causing tumours

12.
    A.   (T)
    B.   (F)   only 15%
    C.   (T)
    D.   (T)
    E.   (F)   growth suppressor factors are anti-oncogenes

13.
    A.   (T)
    B.   (F)   after about 10 days the pH of the uniting fracture increases (alkaline tide)
    C.   (T)
    D.   (F)   woven bone formation occurs whenever there is adequate immobilization
    E.   (T)

14.
    A.   (T)   the metabolite 1-hydroxy-2-naphthylamine is carcinogenic
    B.   (T)
    C.   (F)   bladder cancer never crosses this fascia
    D.   (F)   T3b (see Figure 17a)
    E.   (F)   it has been suggested recently that the presence of squamous metaplasia and β-HCG in the biopsy implies radioresistance

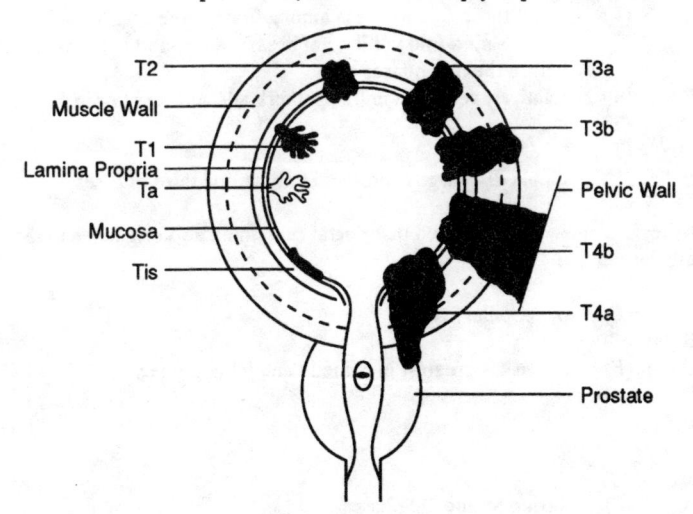

Figure 17a

15.
    A.   (F)   crypt abscesses are more conspicuous in ulcerative colitis
    B.   (F)   a striking finding in ulcerative colitis
    C.   (F)   less frequent in Crohn's disease

	D.	(T)	
	E.	(T)	
16.	A.	(F)	the cartilage of the epiphyseal plate resists the advance of the tumour
	B.	(T)	haematogenous spread
	C.	(T)	
	D.	(F)	commoner in males
	E.	(T)	
17.	A.	(F)	the enlargement of an organ in hyperplasia is due to an increase in the number of its specialized constituent cells
	B.	(F)	this is an important feature of neoplasia
	C.	(T)	
	D.	(T)	
	E.	(T)	
18.	A.	(T)	e.g. closed abdominal trauma, extensive gastro-duodenal surgery
	B.	(F)	appear as small yellow-white nodules of pasty material
	C.	(T)	by producing necrosis of blood vessels
	D.	(F)	by retroperitoneal connective tissue, adherent adjacent viscera and peritoneum of lesser sac
	E.	(F)	calcium combines with fatty acids (liberated by lipase) to form insoluble calcium salts
19.	A.	(F)	about three-fold increase among first degree relatives. The risk reaches nine-fold in bilateral breast cancer and in breast cancer before the menopause
	B.	(T)	relatively very high in the Netherlands and very low in Japan
	C.	(T)	
	D.	(T)	
	E.	(F)	nipple discharge is present in about one third of cases

Note: it is now widely believed that ductal carcinoma also originates in the lobular ductule

20.	A.	(F)	the papillary type
	B.	(T)	
	C.	(F)	the risk is greatest in comedo and lobular types
	D.		
	E.		

21.	A.	(F)	during M and G2 phases
	B.	(T)	
	C.	(F)	they are active synthesizing RNA and proteins
	D.	(F)	this is true of malignant tumours
	E.	(F)	this is true of experimental tumours

GENERAL AND SYSTEMIC PATHOLOGY

22.
- A. (F) total body sodium is usually normal
- B. (F) osmolality decreases due to dilution
- C. (T) dilutional
- D. (T)
- E. (T)

23.
- A. (T)
- B. (T)
- C. (F)
- D. (T)
- E. (F)

24.
- A. (F) 5HT is usually inactivated in the liver by an amine-oxidase
- B. (F) this is rare. Ileal carcinoids commonly cause the syndrome
- C. (F) the right side is more commonly affected. This is due to the pulmonary role in inactivating some secretions of the tumour, e.g. 5HT
- D. (T) diarrhoea and flushing may also be seen
- E. (T) this is a metabolite of 5HT

25.
- A. (F) they are usually solitary, averaging 1.5 cm in diameter, pale brown in colour
- B. (F) see the diagram below
- C. (T) diabetes mellitus is associated with increased cholesterol concentration (See Figure 18)
- D. (T) a shell of calcium may be deposited on the surface of the stone
- E. (F) bile pigment stones may complicate chronic haemolytic anaemias

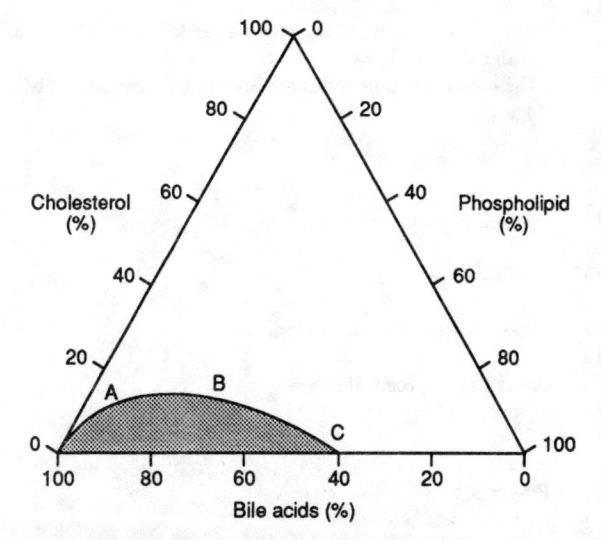

Figure 18 Bile samples above the line ABC are supersaturated with cholesterol

26.
- A. (F) human papilloma virus (HPV) has been implicated
- B. (F)
- C. (F)
- D. (T)
- E. (T)

27.
- A. (T)
- B. (F)
- C. (T)
- D. (F) rectum and appendix are the commonest sites
- E. (F) on or near the lesser curvature

28.
- A. (T)
- B. (F) polypoid carcinoma is associated with a better prognosis
- C. (F) in malignant gastric ulcers, the mucosal folds are interrupted toward the crater
- D. (T)
- E. (T)

29.
- A. (T) ten year survival is approximately 87%
- B. (F) usually there are no psammoma bodies in follicular carcinoma
- C. (F) this is a very rare occurrence. In contrast to that, papillary carcinoma commonly metastasizes to neck lymph nodes
- D. (T)
- E. (F) differentiation of C-cells is a feature of medullary carcinoma

30.
- A. (T)
- B. (T)
- C. (T)
- D. (F) Duke never used 'stage D'. This was added to the classification by others
- E. (F) if the regional lymph nodes are involved the carcinoma will be stage C

31.
- A. (F)
- B. (F)
- C. (T)
- D. (F)
- E. (T)

32.
- A. (F) it has a better prognosis in females
- B. (T)
- C. (F) this is a poor prognostic sign
- D. (F)
- E. (F)

33.
- A. (F) F:M = 3:2
- B. (F)
- C. (T)
- D. (T) a posterior communicating artery aneurysm may produce this palsy by compression
- E. (T)

34.
- A. (T)
- B. (F) there is no disruption
- C. (F) if the wound is contaminated
- D. (F)
- E. (T)

35.
- A. (T)
- B. (T)
- C. (T)
- D. (T)
- E. (F) this usually causes a non-communicating hydrocephalus

36.
- A. (T) less antigen is removed from the portal blood by the diseased liver
- B. (T)
- C. (T) ammonia plays an important part in its causation
- D. (F) this factor is synthesized by the vascular endothelium
- E. (F) cholesterol is synthesized in the liver

37.
- A. (T) and from bone marrow
- B. (F) within 48 hours
- C. (F) only in a small proportion of cases
- D. (T)
- E. (F) may cause haemorrhages in the dermis but not pyoderma gangrenosum

38.
- A. (T)
- B. (F)
- C. (T)
- D. (T) e.g. osteomyelitis
- E. (F)

39.
- A. (T)
- B. (T) this impairs the blood supply
- C. (T)
- D. (T)
- E. (F) this has been shown to be beneficial to wound healing

Microbiology

1. **With respect to tetanus complicating a traumatic wound**

    A. *Clostridium tetani* travels via the nerves to the anterior horn cells in the spinal cord
    B. the tetanospasmin component of the exotoxin acts on synapses to inhibit the normal inhibitory control of motor nerve impulses
    C. the diagnosis is usually made relying on microbiological findings
    D. the patient should be given large doses of antitoxin intravenously
    E. a positive Nagler reaction may identify the presence of *Clostridium tetani* in the wound exudate

2. **Acute osteomyelitis**

    A. is commonest in children under 10 years old
    B. *Haemophilus influenzae* is the responsible pathogen in most cases
    C. blood cultures are rarely positive
    D. usually occurs due to a direct spread of bacteria from a neighbouring septic focus or a penetrating wound
    E. appropriate antibiotic treatment is usually effective

3. **Pseudo-membranous colitis**

    A. is a recognized side-effect of clindamycin
    B. is due to colonization of the colon by *Clostridium perfringens*
    C. procto-sigmoidoscopy is a useful investigation
    D. the microbiologist may make the diagnosis by demonstrating a positive Nagler reaction
    E. aminoglycosides are an effective therapy

4. **The following statements concern some parasitic infestations of surgical importance**

    A. hydatid disease is usually caused by *Entamoeba histolytica*
    B. hydatid disease of the liver most commonly involves the right lobe
    C. a palpable mass in the right iliac fossa is a recognized complication of intestinal amoebiasis
    D. amoebic abscess of the liver can be treated with metronidazole
    E. schistosomiasis of the urinary tract is usually caused by *Schistosoma japonicum*

5. Hepatitis B

- A. the core of the virus contains double stranded DNA
- B. the presence of antibody to e antigen (anti-HBe) correlates with a low infectivity
- C. surface antigen is usually positive in patients with chronic active hepatitis
- D. is the commonest form of hepatitis complicating blood transfusions in the UK
- E. infection can only be transmitted through innoculation

6. The identifying criteria of *Staphylococcus aureus* causing a post-operative wound infection include

- A. coagulase positive
- B. phosphatase negative
- C. fermentation of mannitol
- D. fluorescent greenish appearance of colonies
- E. serology by identification of Lancefield groups

7. *Actinomyces israeli*

- A. are true bacteria
- B. are strict aerobes
- C. cause a chronic granulomatous infection with pus discharges containing yellow-brown sulphur granules
- D. the ileo-caecal region is the commonest site of involvement in actinomycosis
- E. are usually sensitive to penicillin

8. The following organisms are recognized causes of diarrhoea in man

- A. *Staphylococcus aureus*
- B. *Yersinia pseudotuberculosis*
- C. *Streptococcus dysgalactiae*
- D. *Staphylococcus epidermidis*
- E. *Clostridium perfringens*

9. The gastro-intestinal complications of AIDS include

- A. colitis due to cytomegalovirus
- B. diarrhoea and superficial ulcers due to *Mycobacterium avium intracellulare*
- C. chronic perianal herpes simplex
- D. salmonella entero-colitis
- E. Kaposi sarcoma

10. Tuberculosis

   A. the primary complex may involve the tonsils with cervical adenitis
   B. a positive Mantoux test means complete protection against tuberculosis
   C. direct microscopy of a smear stained by the auramine method confirms the diagnosis in most cases
   D. the diagnosis of tuberculous peritonitis is usually made on the basis of clinical examination and positive blood cultures
   E. streptomycin remains the drug of choice

11. Cefuroxime is active against

   A. *Staphylococcus aureus*
   B. *Streptococcus pyogenes*
   C. *Streptococcus faecalis*
   D. *Pseudomonas aeruginosa*
   E. *Bacteroides fragilis*

12. The pathophysiological effects of endotoxins include

   A. initial leukopenia
   B. release of interleukin 1
   C. inhibition of Hageman factor
   D. activation of the alternative complement pathway
   E. stimulation of platelet aggregation

13. With respect to some surgically important infections

   A. osteomyelitis is a recognized complication of furuncles
   B. carbuncles are usually caused by *Streptococcus pyogenes*
   C. erysipelas is usually due to *Erysipelothrix rhusiopathiae*
   D. acute orchitis may be due to *Neisseria gonorrhoeae*
   E. the production of coagulase by *Streptococcus pyogenes* explains its invasiveness in cellulitis

14. With respect to some fungi and fungal infections

   A. the antibody response to candida is reduced in chronic mucocutaneous candidiasis
   B. *Cryptococcus neoformans* has a capsule which can be demonstrated in India ink
   C. in aspergilloma *Aspergillus fumigatus* grows in an existing lung cavity to form a ball of mycelium
   D. oral griseofulvin is the treatment of choice for invasive aspergillosis
   E. coccidioidomycosis is due to a dimorphic fungus

15. Mumps

- A. is due to a DNA virus
- B. epididymoorchitis occurs in about 30% of patients who develop mumps after puberty
- C. melanosis coli is a recognized complication
- D. parotid glands are more frequently involved than the submandibular glands
- E. live attenuated mumps virus vaccine is usually used in prevention

16. *Staphylococcus aureus* is usually responsible for abscess formation in the following sites

- A. appendix
- B. axilla
- C. finger pulp
- D. ischio-rectal regions
- E. breast

17. *Streptococcus pyogenes*, causing an open wound infection, is usually sensitive to

- A. erythromycin
- B. polymyxin
- C. vancomycin
- D. nalidixic acid
- E. penicillin

18. With respect to a sample of intra-abdominal pus the microbiologist

- A. usually examines a smear of the sample under the microscope
- B. does not usually re-incubate the plate cultures if they are sterile after overnight incubation
- C. may need to perform Weil–Felix agglutination test
- D. routinely seeds the specimen on two blood agar plates (one incubated aerobically plus CO_2 and the other anaerobically plus CO_2) and a cooked meat broth
- E. may perform gas–liquid chromatography

19. The following statements concern a sputum sample from a patient with a possible respiratory tract infection

A. the sample should always be processed, even if it is 36 hours old
B. the microbiologist may liquefy and dilute the specimen to get better results
C. an optochin sensitivity test is indicated if cultures yield a moderate growth of α-haemolytic Gram-positive cocci
D. the microbiologist should report the result of antibiotic sensitivity tests even if the cultures yielded a scanty mixed growth only
E. if the patient has Legionnaire's disease, the responsible *Legionella pneumophilia* can be easily cultured from the specimen

20. The following bacteria may cause gas gangrene

A. *Clostridium septicum*
B. *Clostridium histolyticum*
C. *Staphylococcus aureus*
D. *Listeria monocytogenes*
E. *Clostridium novyi (oedematiens)*

21. In hospitals, *Pseudomonas aeruginosa* may cause

A. urinary tract infection
B. meningitis
C. osteomyelitis
D. wound infection
E. conjunctivitis

22. The following antimicrobials are active against *Bacteroides fragilis*

A. gentamicin
B. metronidazole
C. ampicillin
D. clindamycin
E. cefuroxime

23. *Staphylococcus aureus*

A. possesses leukocidins
B. is resistant to phagocytosis by polymorphonuclear leukocytes
C. is usually responsible for carbuncles
D. phage type III is the commonest cause of boils
E. is usually sensitive to fusidic acid

24. The following statements are correct

A. vancomycin is well absorbed from the gut
B. vancomycin and penicillin inhibit bacterial cell wall synthesis by the same mechanism
C. metronidazole readily crosses the blood–brain barrier
D. clindamycin is active against gastrointestinal *Bacteroides fragilis*
E. sulphonamides readily cross the blood–brain barrier

25. The following antimicrobials act by inhibiting the cell wall synthesis of the microbe

A. cefuroxime
B. vancomycin
C. erythromycin
D. gentamicin
E. amphotericin B

Answers

1. A. (F) *Clostridium tetani* does not spread beyond the wound, but the exotoxin does
   B. (T)
   C. (F) the diagnosis is usually clinical
   D. (T) to neutralize toxin
   E. (F) this is an identification for *Clostridium perfringens*

2. A. (T)
   B. (F) *Staphylococcus aureus* accounts for more than 75% of cases
   C. (F) positive in a high proportion of cases
   D. (F) (haematogenous spread)
   E. (T) must be continued for several weeks

3. A. (T)
   B. (F) *Clostridum difficile* is the causative bacteria
   C. (T) pseudomembranous plaques may be seen; these should be biopsied
   D. (F) by demonstrating the cytotoxic effect of toxin in a faecal filtrate and the neutralization of the toxin by specific antiserum
   E. (F) clostridia are resistant to aminoglycosides

4. A. (F) by *Echinococcus* (*E. granulosus* or *E. multilocularis*)
   B. (T)
   C. (F) amoebic granuloma
   D. (T) aspiration may be needed
   E. (F) usually caused by *Schistosoma haematobium*

5.
- A. (T)
- B. (T)
- C. (F)
- D. (F) non-A non-B hepatitis (hepatitis C) is the commonest
- E. (F)

6.
- A. (T)
- B. (F) phosphatase positive
- C. (T)
- D. (F) the colonies are typically golden, but pigmentation ranges from orange to white
- E. (F) this applies to a streptococcus

7.
- A. (T)
- B. (F) strict anaerobes
- C. (T)
- D. (F) the ileo-caecal region is involved in about 20% of cases. Cervico-facial actinomycosis is the commonest, accounting for about 65% of cases
- E. (T)

8.
- A. (T)
- B. (T)
- C. (F)
- D. (F)
- E. (T)

9. All true.
A, B, C and D are examples of opportunistic infections

10.
- A. (T)
- B. (F) a positive test reflects a degree of immunity
- C. (T)
- D. (F) usually made at laparotomy
- E. (F) this has been replaced by less toxic drugs, e.g. isoniazid, rifampicin, ethambutol, etc

11.
- A. (T)
- B. (T)
- C. (F)
- D. (F)
- E. (F)

12.
- A. (T)
- B. (T) causing fever
- C. (F)
- D. (T)
- E. (T)

See Figure 19

MICROBIOLOGY

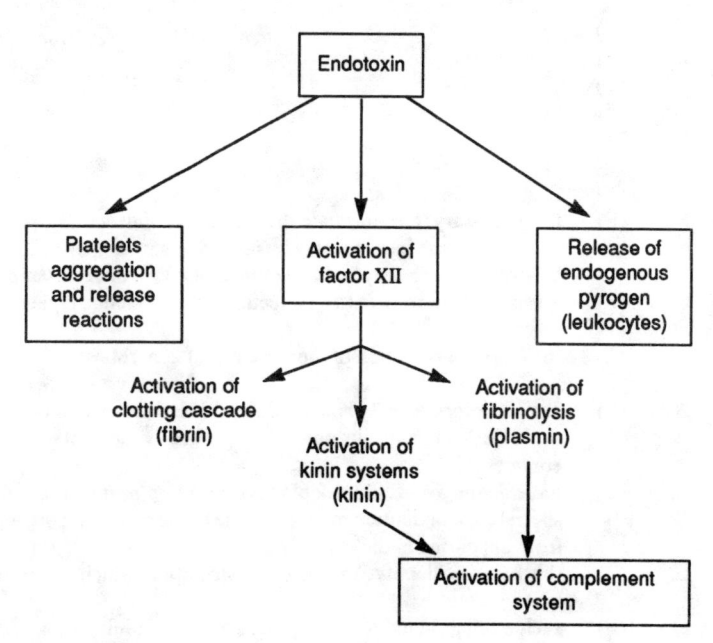

```
                    ┌─────────────┐
                    │  Endotoxin  │
                    └─────────────┘
           ↙               ↓               ↘
┌──────────────┐  ┌──────────────┐  ┌──────────────┐
│   Platelets  │  │ Activation of│  │   Release of │
│  aggregation │  │  factor XII  │  │  endogenous  │
│  and release │  │              │  │    pyrogen   │
│   reactions  │  │              │  │ (leukocytes) │
└──────────────┘  └──────────────┘  └──────────────┘
          ↙           ↓           ↘
  Activation of                   Activation of
 clotting cascade               fibrinolysis
     (fibrin)                     (plasmin)
                Activation of
               kinin systems
                   (kinin)
                      ↘             ↓
                    ┌──────────────────────────┐
                    │ Activation of complement │
                    │         system           │
                    └──────────────────────────┘
```

Figure 19

13.
- A. (T)
- B. (F) by *Staphylococcus aureus*
- C. (F) usually due to streptococci
- D. (T)
- E. (F) the production of hyaluronidase and streptokinase explains the invasiveness

14.
- A. (F) T-cell mediated immunity is impaired, but the antibody response is normal
- B. (T)
- C. (T)
- D. (F) intravenous amphotericin B
- E. (T)

15.
- A. (F) an RNA paramyxovirus
- B. (T)
- C. (F) this may complicate purgative abuse
- D. (T)
- E. (T)

16.
- A. (F) faecal flora, *Streptococcus milleri*
- B. (T)
- C. (T) through a penetrating wound
- D. (F) faecal flora from the rectum
- E. (T)

17.
- A. (T)
- B. (F)
- C. (T)
- D. (F)
- E. (T)

18.
- A. (T) this is very important
- B. (F) it is necessary to re-incubate the plates for a further day, otherwise some bacteria may be missed, e.g. non-sporing anaerobes which may be present in about 30% of such samples
- C. (F) this is relevant to rickettsial infections, e.g. epidemic typhus
- D. (T)
- E. (T) for rapid confirmation of the presence of anaerobes

19.
- A. (F) samples more than 24 hours old should be discarded in order to avoid misleading results due to overgrowth of the contaminating commensals
- B. (T) liquefaction avoids the risk of choosing a non-purulent part of the specimen, and dilution may prevent the contaminating organisms from appearing in the cultures
- C. (T) this helps to identify *Streptococcus pneumonia* which is sensitive to it
- D. (F) such a thing should not be reported as the administration of antibiotics active against the normal flora may render these organisms resistant to the antibiotic
- E. (F) this organism may be seen in the specimen (Gram-negative pleomorphic coccobacillus), but it is difficult to culture

20.
- A. (T)
- B. (T)
- C. (F)
- D. (F)
- E. (T)

21. All true. Note: it is difficult to control hospital infections due to this organism because of its ability to grow in solutions used for treatment and its natural resistance to many antimicrobials

22.
- A. (F)
- B. (T)
- C. (F)
- D. (T)
- E. (F)

23.
- A. (T)
- B. (F) it is readily phagocytosed by these cells, but the polymorphs are killed after phagocytosis
- C. (T)
- D. (F) mainly *Staphylococcus aureus* phage type I and II
- E. (T)

24.
	A.	(F)	this explains its efficacy in pseudomembranous colitis
	B.	(F)	the mechanisms of inhibition are different
	C.	(T)	it may be of value in the treatment of non-traumatic cerebral abscess
	D.	(T)	
	E.	(T)	

25.
	A.	(T)	
	B.	(T)	
	C.	(F)	inhibits protein synthesis in ribosomes
	D.	(F)	the same as in C
	E.	(F)	interferes with the barrier function of the cell membrane

Clinical Immunology

1. **With regard to cadaveric kidney transplantation**

    A. CD4 and CD8 cells mediate the acute rejection of transplantation
    B. DRw6-negative grafts do better than DRw6-positive ones
    C. multiple blood transfusions prior to grafting increase graft rejection
    D. the five-year survival rate of the transplanted kidney is better for one DR mismatch than for two DR mismatches
    E. cyclosporin A is a useful anti-rejection therapy

2. **The statements below concern organ transplantation**

    A. the three-year survival of heart transplants with single DR mismatches is about 90% nowadays
    B. cyclosporin A has not improved the survival figures for cardiac transplantation
    C. only about 25% of patients with liver transplants for hepatic cancer have had recurrence of their tumour within one year
    D. pancreas allografts have a better one-year survival than cardiac allografts
    E. the recipient marrow and lymphoid systems are destroyed by chemotherapy and/or irradiation prior to bone marrow transplantation

3. **The following are examples of antibody-dependent cytotoxic hypersensitivity (type II)**

    A. hyperthyroidism in Graves' disease
    B. haemolytic anaemia due to *Mycoplasma pneumoniae*
    C. haemolysis following blood transfusion
    D. the main mechanism mediating acute early rejection of a transplanted kidney
    E. hyperacute rejection of a transplanted kidney

4. **With regard to cell-mediated (type IV) hypersensitivity reaction**

    A. CD8 cells recognize antigen in conjunction with class II molecules
    B. the reaction is seen in the rejection of a transplanted kidney
    C. the reaction takes 4–10 hours to develop
    D. sensitized CD4 cells produce lymphokines which help macrophages to kill intracellular parasites
    E. cell mediated immunity has been implicated in the protection against some cancers

CLINICAL IMMUNOLOGY

5. Cell mediated (type IV/delayed hypersensitivity) reactions are

   A. dependent on complement
   B. independent of antibody
   C. dependent on T-lymphocytes
   D. usually increased in AIDS patients
   E. responsible for autoimmune haemolytic anaemia

6. The statements below concern hypersensitivity reactions

   A. anaphylactic hypersensitivity (type I) depends on the reaction of antigen with specific IgE antibody bound to the mast cell
   B. complex mediated hypersensitivity (type III) does not involve complement
   C. the formation of chronic granulomata is an example of type IV (delayed hypersensitivity) reactions
   D. steroids are effective against late type I (anaphylactic) reaction
   E. pernicious anaemia is an example of type II hypersensitivity

7. With respect to interleukin-2 (IL-2) and interferons

   A. IL-2 is secreted by stimulated CD4 cells
   B. therapy with lymphokine activated cells and IL-2 produces a good response rate in the treatment of sarcomas
   C. IL-2 acts mainly on resting cells prior to polyclonal activation
   D. α-interferon inhibits viral activation and stimulates NK cells
   E. interferons have an anti-proliferative function

8. Considering a patient with AIDS

   A. the CD4 molecule on helper inducer T cells enabled the AIDS virus to bind and to infect lymphocytes
   B. there is a fall in the CD8:CD4 ratio in the peripheral blood
   C. the patient may have β-lymphocytes which are polyclonally activated
   D. almost all the surviving peripheral CD4 cells are positive for the viral genome
   E. the susceptibility to cytomegalovirus (CMV) infection is due to failure to produce CMV specific cytotoxic T cells

9. With respect to AIDS

   A. the first antibodies to appear after infection are directed to core proteins
   B. skin tests to common antigens are usually suppressed
   C. cyclosporin-A inhibits the reverse transcriptase enzyme of the virus
   D. soluble CD4 molecules bind to HIV and block its infectivity
   E. the diagnosis is usually confirmed by positive isolation of HIV-I

Answers

1.
- A. (T)
- B. (F) DRw6-positive grafts do better
- C. (F) have a beneficial effect
- D. (T)
- E. (T)

2.
- A. (T)
- B. (F)
- C. (F) about 75% have had recurrence
- D. (F) 40% for pancreas and 85% for heart
- E. (T)

3.
- A. (F) this is an example of type V hypersensitivity (stimulatory)
- B. (T)
- C. (T)
- D. (F) this appears to be cell mediated hypersensitivity through T-lymphocytes
- E. (T)

4.
- A. (F) in conjunction with class I molecules
- B. (T)
- C. (F) 12–24 hours
- D. (T)
- E. (T)

5.
- A. (F) independent of complement
- B. (T)
- C. (T)
- D. (F) (decreased)
- E. (F) autoimmune haemolytic anaemia is an example of type II hypersensitivity

6.
- A. (T)
- B. (F)
- C. (T) due to persisting antigen
- D. (T)
- E. (T)

7.
- A. (T)
- B. (F) sarcomas are rather resistant. Colo-rectal cancer, melanomas and renal carcinomas respond better
- C. (F) IL-2 receptors are not present on such cells
- D. (T)
- E. (T)

8.
A. (T)
B. (F) there is a fall in the T4:T8 not T8:T4 ratio
C. (T) and hypergammaglobulinaemia
D. (F) only 1 in 10^4 to 1 in 10^5 are positive for the viral genome
E. (T)

9.
A. (F) antibodies directed against the p110 envelope glycoprotein appear first
B. (T) due to depressed cell mediated immunity
C. (F)
D. (T)
E. (F) by demonstrating viral antibodies to ELISA or immunoblotting

Haematology

1. **With respect to cross-matching of blood for transfusion**

    A. the patient's serum is screened for atypical IgM antibodies at 37°C using saline techniques
    B. direct Coombs' test is performed to detect antibodies in the patient against donor red blood cells
    C. the erythrocytes from each donor unit are tested against the patient's serum at 37°C to detect IgG antibodies
    D. the cross-match usually takes about 1 hour
    E. if no time is allowed for cross-matching, group O rhesus positive blood should be transfused

2. **With respect to Hodgkin's disease**

    A. lymphocyte predominant histology is associated with the best prognosis
    B. the inguinal region is the commonest site for superficial lymphadenopathy at presentation
    C. the presence of Reed–Sternberg cells is essential to making the diagnosis
    D. the disease does not involve non-lymphatic tissue
    E. cyclical chemotherapy is the treatment of choice in patients with stage I disease

3. **With respect to a patient with iron deficiency anaemia due to a chronic peptic ulcer, the laboratory findings include**

    A. normal ferritin
    B. low serum iron
    C. complete absence of iron from macrophages in bone marrow
    D. low total iron binding capacity (TIBC)
    E. decreased mean corpuscular volume (MCV)

4. **The following laboratory results are consistent with a diagnosis of disseminated intravascular coagulation (DIC) in a surgical patient who develops a gram-negative septicaemia**

    A. prolonged thrombin time
    B. low platelet count
    C. elevated levels of fibrinogen degradation products in serum
    D. elevated fibrinogen levels in serum
    E. reduced factor VIII activity

5. Idiopathic thrombocytopenic purpura (ITP)

A. an auto-antibody can be demonstrated in about 70% of subjects
B. the auto-antibody cannot cross the placenta
C. the majority of cases respond temporarily to steroids (up to 3 mg/kg of prednisone)
D. when a patient with ITP is transfused with platelets, the transfused platelets survive longer than the patient's own platelets
E. the intravenous administration of high dose IgG is a recognized treatment modality

6. The bleeding time may be prolonged in the following

A. von Willebrand's disease
B. vitamin K deficiency
C. haemophilia A
D. idiopathic thrombocytopenic purpura
E. liver disease

7. With respect to haemophilia A

A. the prothrombin time (PT) is prolonged
B. the gene coding for the deficient factor is located on the long arm of the X chromosome
C. the prenatal diagnosis by DNA analysis is now possible
D. the gene coding for the deficient factor has been cloned
E. the level of the protein VIII R:Ag is characteristically low

8. The partial thromboplastin time with kaolin (PTTK) is usually prolonged in

A. haemophilia
B. von Willebrand's disease
C. vitamin K deficiency
D. idiopathic thrombocytopenic purpura
E. a patient who is fully heparinized

9. Recognized consequences of blood transfusion include

A. haemoglobinuria
B. hypothermia
C. hyperkalaemia
D. air embolism
E. amoebiasis

10. The following statements refer to blood groups and transfusion of blood products

    A.   patients of group O possess anti-A and anti-B antibodies in their serum
    B.   the possession of antigen d (rather than antigen D) makes the subject rhesus positive (Rh^+)
    C.   anti-D antibodies are naturally occurring antibodies
    D.   cryoprecipitate contains all coagulation factors
    E.   HLA-antibodies are an important cause of febrile transfusion reactions

11. The following are recognized causes of splenomegaly

    A.   iron deficiency anaemia
    B.   schistosomiasis
    C.   primary thrombocytopaenia
    D.   portal hypertension
    E.   metastatic tumour

Answers

1.   A. (F) the detection of IgM antibodies (cold) is carried out at room temperature
      B. (F) the indirect Coombs' test is used for this purpose
      C. (T)
      D. (T)
      E. (F) group O rhesus negative blood should be transfused

2.   A. (T)
      B. (F) the cervical lymph nodes are most commonly involved at presentation
      C. (T)
      D. (F) the involvement of non-lymphatic tissue (e.g. skin, lung, brain, etc.) usually occurs late
      E. (F) radiotherapy is the treatment of choice for stages I and II

3.   A. (F) the ferritin is usually reduced
      B. (T)
      C. (T)
      D. (F) the TIBC rises as the saturation decreases due to iron deficiency
      E. (T)

4.   A. (T)
      B. (T)
      C. (T)
      D. (F) there is fibrinogen deficiency
      E. (T)

5.
A.	(T)	
B.	(F)	the antibody (IgG) can cross the placenta, causing neonatal thrombocytopenia
C.	(T)	then splenoctomy can be safely performed. Following splenoctomy the long-term remission rate is about 70% of cases
D.	(F)	due to the presence of the antibody
E.	(T)	

6.
A.	(T)	platelet function is impaired
B.	(F)	
C.	(F)	
D.	(T)	
E.	(T)	this may cause platelet dysfunction

7.
A.	(F)	PT is normal
B.	(T)	X-linked inheritance
C.	(T)	after chorionic villus sampling
D.	(T)	
E.	(F)	the level of VIII:C is low (coagulant activity)

8.
A.	(T)
B.	(T)
C.	(T)
D.	(F)
E.	(T)

Note. PTTK is sensitive to factors in the intrinsic and common pathways

9.
A.	(T)
B.	(T)
C.	(T)
D.	(T)
E.	(F)

10.
A.	(T)	
B.	(F)	the possession of the D antigen makes the subject Rh$^+$
C.	(F)	these antibodies nearly always arise after immunization by transfusion or pregnancy
D.	(F)	cryoprecipitate contains factor VIII and fibrinogen. Fresh frozen plasma (FFP) contains all coagulation factors
E.	(T)	

11.
A.	(T)	
B.	(T)	
C.	(T)	
D.	(T)	
E.	(T)	this is surprisingly rare

Clinical Chemistry

1. In a 60-year-old man with the syndrome of inappropriate ADH secretion (due to a bronchial neoplasm) the following results are strongly consistent with the diagnosis

    A. serum sodium 115 mmol/L
    B. urine osmolality 360 mmol/kg
    C. serum osmolality 300 mmol/kg
    D. a biochemical response to fluid restriction
    E. urine sodium 15 mmol/L

2. The serum potassium of a 60-year-old lady was found to be 2.2 mmol/L. The following conditions may explain this abnormal result

    A. frusemide therapy
    B. Addison's disease (not associated with hypovolaemic shock)
    C. villous adenoma of the rectum
    D. diarrhoea
    E. untreated diabetic keto-acidosis

3. The following results are very compatible with a diagnosis of acute pre-renal failure in a surgical patient

    A. urine sodium concentration 50 mmol/L
    B. ratio of urine to serum urea concentration of 2:1
    C. serum potassium 6.0 mmol/L
    D. blood pressure 85/50
    E. blood pH 7.30

4. Common consequences of chronic renal failure include

    A. metabolic acidosis
    B. hypercalcaemia
    C. normochromic normocytic anaemia
    D. hypophosphataemia
    E. decreased insulin requirements in an insulin dependent diabetic patient

5. Hyperkalaemia is usually a feature of

    A. acute renal failure
    B. chronic renal failure
    C. pyloric stenosis
    D. Conn's syndrome
    E. inappropriate ADH secretion

6. A 70-year-old man was admitted to hospital with breathlessness. Arterial blood analysis was performed: PCO_2 9.3, pH 7.32 (HCO_3^-) 34

   A. the results suggest an acute respiratory acidosis
   B. the results indicate that there is a renal compensation to a respiratory acidosis
   C. this patient may have a co-existing metabolic acidosis
   D. the results are compatible with a diagnosis of an exacerbation of chronic obstructive airways disease
   E. this patient can be safely given oxygen at a high concentration

7. Gastric acid secretion and serum gastrin are simultaneously elevated in

   A. pernicious anaemia
   B. Zollinger–Ellison syndrome
   C. after vagotomy
   D. hypersecretion of gastrin by antral G-cells
   E. atrophic gastritis

8. Serum alkaline phosphatase is usually greater than five times the upper limit of normal (5 × ULN) in the following

   A. Paget's disease of bone
   B. uncomplicated osteoporosis
   C. healing fractures
   D. extra-hepatic cholestasis
   E. hypothyroidism

9. The causes of hyperprolactinaemia include

   A. pregnancy
   B. pituitary stalk secretion
   C. chronic renal failure
   D. dopamine agonists
   E. hypothyroidism

10. During the first 24 hours following uncomplicated hemicolectomy

    A. urinary potassium excretion increases
    B. urinary sodium excretion increases
    C. urine osmolality decreases
    D. the patient is in negative nitrogen balance
    E. catecholamines output by the adrenal medulla decreases

11. The following tumour markers and malignancies are correctly paired

A. calcitonin – some cases of breast carcinoma
B. α-fetoprotein – hepatocellular carcinoma
C. α-fetoprotein – colo-rectal cancer
D. carcino-embryonic antigen (CEA) – testicular teratomas
E. human chorionic gonadotrophin (HCG) – choriocarcinoma

12. With respect to Cushing's syndrome

A. adrenal carcinoma is a recognized cause
B. if there is a significant suppression of cortisol secretion in response to a low dose of dexamethasone the diagnosis is Cushing's disease
C. there is impairment of wound healing
D. secretion of ACTH by the pituitary is increased in ectopic ACTH secretion
E. trans-sphenoidal hypophysectomy is a treatment modality for Cushing's disease

13. The causes of hypocalcaemia include

A. thyroidectomy
B. acute pancreatitis
C. milk–alkali syndrome
D. sarcoidosis
E. magnesium deficiency

14. The following are recognized causes of hypercalcaemia

A. renal transplantation
B. thiazide diuretics
C. frusemide administration in a healthy subject
D. thyrotoxicosis
E. hypoparathyroidism

15. Failure to excrete a water load (1 litre taken orally) is a feature of

A. adrenocortical insufficiency
B. loss of hypothalamic osmotic receptors
C. cranial diabetes insipidus
D. hepatic failure
E. hyperglycaemia

CLINICAL CHEMISTRY

Answers

1. A. (T) dilutional hyponatraemia
   B. (T) concentrated urine
   C. (F) the serum osmolality is usually decreased in this syndrome (i.e. <280 mmol/kg)
   D. (T)
   E. (F) there is usually a continued sodium loss in urine (>20 mmol/L). This is due to the fact that the plasma volume is maintained by water retention and hence there is no hypovolaemic stimulus to aldosterone secretion

2. A. (T)
   B. (F) due to mineralo-cortical deficiency
   C. (T) these tumours may secrete excessive potassium
   D. (T)
   E. (F) this usually causes hyperkalaemia which is due to both haemoconcentration from fluid loss and acidosis

3. A. (F) in pre-renal failure (Na^+) in urine is usually less than 20 mmol/L. This is due to increased secretion of aldosterone
   B. (F) (urea) urine: (urea) serum is usually greater than 10
   C. (T) this is due to decreased delivery of Na^+ to the distal tubule. See A
   D. (T) circulatory insufficiency is the usual cause of acute pre-renal failure
   E. (T) a metabolic acidosis ensues as the excretion of H^+ is reduced. See A

4. A. (T)
   B. (F) hypocalcaemia usually ensues
   C. (T) due to depression of bone marrow by accumulated toxins and to decreased erythropoietin synthesis by the unhealthy kidney
   D. (F) hyperphosphataemia ensues
   E. (T) due to the fact that insulin is metabolized in the kidneys

5. A. (T)
   B. (T)
   C. (F) hypokalaemia ensues due to loss of K^+ in the vomitus and to preservation of Na^+ (and water) at the expense of K^+ by the kidneys
   D. (F) this is primary hyperaldosteronism. Aldosterone promotes sodium reabsorption and potassium secretion in the distal convoluted tubule and collecting ducts of the kidney
   E. (F) hypokalaemia is a feature

6. A. (F) the high concentration of bicarbonate suggests that there is renal compensation (which usually takes several days to become established) in response to a chronic respiratory acidosis
   B. (T) See A

	C.	(F)	[HCO$_3^-$] is elevated
	D.	(T)	
	E.	(F)	in chronic CO$_2$ retention hypoxia becomes the main stimulus to the respiratory drive: therefore the abolition of such a stimulus can be dangerous
7.	A.	(F)	absolute achlorhydria is present
	B.	(T)	
	C.	(F)	gastric acid secretion is reduced
	D.	(T)	
	E.	(F)	this may cause achlorhydria
8.	A.	(T)	
	B.	(F)	the level is normal
	C.	(F)	serum alkaline phosphatase is increased in this condition, although it is usually <5 × ULN
	D.	(T)	
	E.	(F)	the level may be decreased
9.	A.	(T)	
	B.	(T)	this may interrupt the inhibitory control
	C.	(T)	
	D.	(F)	dopamine agonists such as bromocriptine tend to lower prolactin levels
	E.	(T)	
10.	A.	(T)	tissue damage and increased aldosterone contribute to this
	B.	(F)	decreases. Increased aldosterone contributes to this
	C.	(F)	increases due to increased excretion of urea and other nitrogenous compounds. Also more water is reabsorbed under the influence of increased ADH
	D.	(T)	
	E.	(F)	increases
11.	A.	(T)	ectopic secretion
	B.	(T)	high serum levels are found in about 70% of cases
	C.	(F)	CEA has been used as a marker, although its value is doubtful
	D.	(F)	α-FP and HCG are markers for testicular teratomas
	E.	(T)	
12.	A.	(T)	
	B.	(F)	in Cushing's disease there is a response to the high dose but not to the low dose
	C.	(T)	
	D.	(F)	the pituitary ACTH secretion is decreased due to negative feedback by excessive cortisol
	E.	(T)	this has been recently re-introduced
13.	A.	(T)	the parathyroid glands may be inadvertently removed
	B.	(T)	the lipase released from the inflamed organ liberates free fatty

CLINICAL CHEMISTRY

	C.	(F)	acids which in turn bind to calcium causing hypocalcaemia this is an uncommon cause of hypocalcaemia
	D.	(F)	there is 1-hydroxylation of 25-hydroxycholecalciferol by the macrophages causing hypercalcaemia as a result
	E.	(T)	
14.	A.	(T)	tertiary hyperparathyroidism
	B.	(T)	decrease renal excretion
	C.	(F)	this promotes renal excretion
	D.	(T)	
	E.	(F)	this causes hypocalcaemia
15.	A.	(T)	
	B.	(T)	this may be seen in neurosurgery, e.g. removal of craniopharyngioma
	C.	(F)	this causes polyuria
	D.	(T)	
	E.	(F)	polyuria may ensue